PUBLIC HEALTH IN THE 21ST CENTURY

# BIOETHICS AND NEGLECTED DISEASES

# PUBLIC HEALTH IN THE 21ST CENTURY

Additional books and e-books in this series can be found
on Nova's website under the Series tab.

PUBLIC HEALTH IN THE 21ST CENTURY

# BIOETHICS AND NEGLECTED DISEASES

MIGUEL KOTTOW

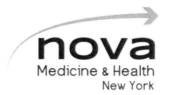

Medicine & Health
New York

Copyright © 2019 by Nova Science Publishers, Inc.

**All rights reserved.** No part of this book may be reproduced, stored in a retrieval system or transmitted in any form or by any means: electronic, electrostatic, magnetic, tape, mechanical photocopying, recording or otherwise without the written permission of the Publisher.

We have partnered with Copyright Clearance Center to make it easy for you to obtain permissions to reuse content from this publication. Simply navigate to this publication's page on Nova's website and locate the "Get Permission" button below the title description. This button is linked directly to the title's permission page on copyright.com. Alternatively, you can visit copyright.com and search by title, ISBN, or ISSN.

For further questions about using the service on copyright.com, please contact:
Copyright Clearance Center
Phone: +1-(978) 750-8400          Fax: +1-(978) 750-4470          E-mail: info@copyright.com.

## NOTICE TO THE READER

The Publisher has taken reasonable care in the preparation of this book, but makes no expressed or implied warranty of any kind and assumes no responsibility for any errors or omissions. No liability is assumed for incidental or consequential damages in connection with or arising out of information contained in this book. The Publisher shall not be liable for any special, consequential, or exemplary damages resulting, in whole or in part, from the readers' use of, or reliance upon, this material. Any parts of this book based on government reports are so indicated and copyright is claimed for those parts to the extent applicable to compilations of such works.

Independent verification should be sought for any data, advice or recommendations contained in this book. In addition, no responsibility is assumed by the Publisher for any injury and/or damage to persons or property arising from any methods, products, instructions, ideas or otherwise contained in this publication.

This publication is designed to provide accurate and authoritative information with regard to the subject matter covered herein. It is sold with the clear understanding that the Publisher is not engaged in rendering legal or any other professional services. If legal or any other expert assistance is required, the services of a competent person should be sought. FROM A DECLARATION OF PARTICIPANTS JOINTLY ADOPTED BY A COMMITTEE OF THE AMERICAN BAR ASSOCIATION AND A COMMITTEE OF PUBLISHERS.

Additional color graphics may be available in the e-book version of this book.

## Library of Congress Cataloging-in-Publication Data

ISBN: 978-1-53615-333-0
Library of Congress Control Number: 2019937814

*Published by Nova Science Publishers, Inc. † New York*

*The almost unsolvable task consists in not being duped by the power of others or by one's own impotence.*

(T. Adorno)

# CONTENTS

| | | |
|---|---|---|
| **Introduction** | | ix |
| **Chapter 1** | Rights and Justice | 1 |
| **Chapter 2** | Medicine in Health and Disease | 35 |
| **Chapter 3** | Strategies of Biomedical Research | 47 |
| **Chapter 4** | Neglected and Rare Diseases | 71 |
| **Chapter 5** | Medical Anthropology for Bioethics | 97 |
| **Chapter 6** | Ethics and Neglected Diseases | 115 |
| **Chapter 7** | Coping with Neglected Populations | 125 |
| **Chapter 8** | Bioethics and Neglected Diseases | 143 |
| **Chapter 9** | Gadfly Bioethics | 171 |
| **References** | | 181 |
| **About the Author** | | 197 |
| **Index** | | 199 |
| **Related Nova Publications** | | 207 |

# INTRODUCTION

Attention to the underprivileged has historically been the turf of socialist political discourses, emerging as cries for the liberation of people living under oppressive dictatorships. After Marxism foundered and ceased to be a political alternative threatening capitalism, the idea of a revolutionary proletariat dissolved into the acceptance that neoliberalism had pursued the conversion of many of the underprivileged into members of a pacified yet avid consumer society, devoid of ethical concerns for a persistent proximal and distant "substratum of outcasts and outsiders, the exploited and persecuted of other races and other colours, the unemployed and the unemployable" as Marcuse wrote in *One-Dimensional Man* (1964).

Rebellious outcries against oppressive dictatorships have lost force, as liberationist efforts are ruthlessly crushed or make true that revolutions devour their own children. International blame and shame are ineffectually showered on rogue states, while lacking self-critical appraisal of their uselessness, unless underpinned by economic sanctions. The latter, often cloaked as "humanitarian aid", wage wars that claim to restore democracy but in fact strategically pursue major economic or military gains.

Without too much concern about the destination of national revenues, and the fact that global and regional income disparities are on the rise, statistics are juggled to favor reaching the opposite conclusion: as the world becomes wealthier, the poor tend to improve their income and, supposedly, their lot. Reality does not substantiate such self-congratulatory optimism.

Globalization has substantially increased resources for healthcare, yet its provision is more unequal than ever, ranging from medicalization-induced overconsumption of medical services and products, to the unchanging statistical fact that one-third of the world population is affected by one or more neglected diseases, that is, conditions that could be prevented or successfully treated with technoscientific resources.

Within this reality, there exist a number of diseases that are so infrequent as to qualify as orphan or rare diseases, mostly of genetic origin causing severe disabilities and life-threatening conditions. Whereas neglected diseases are exacerbated by disgraceful socioeconomic factors, sufferers from rare diseases receive limited biomedical research −at some time they were called non-profitable diseases−. When promising therapeutic agents are presented, they are priced at what many have called outrageous levels that challenge to deplete private, institutional or public funds.

Complex issues can be described, even correctly diagnosed in their problematic nature, but solutions to social Gordian knots are nowhere in sight, except by the swords of dogma and totalitarianism. Imperfect or failing democracies and oppressive political systems are always associated with undercurrents of ethical critique of the present and hopes for a better future. Marginalized from power, ethics has never been a motor of social change; it cannot claim ascendancy, but must doggedly follow a path of persistent coherence. In whichever form the turmoil of social change finally subsides, ethics will be reprimanded for having remained silent even if speaking up would have been no more than a helpless gesture.

In a world where intellectual work is just another commodity hoping to survive in the market economy of knowledge, there seems little point in repeatedly going over structural realities potently causing and sustaining chronic global maladies such as injustice and healthcare inequity, impervious to any sign of will or power to improve the lot of the unfortunate. Be that as it may, ethics cannot be excused from unveiling neglect, and revealing unrecognized wretched human beings.

*Introduction* xi

Issues and problems concerning healthcare inequities, neglected populations, and unattended rare diseases, are here taken up without undue hopes of influence, yet believing in the duty that man-made harms and wrongs should be exposed. At the very least, this presentation aims at puncturing the self-congratulatory conviction that globalization and neoliberalism are compatible with comprehensive fairness and wellbeing for all, insistently pretending that global negativities are being attended to, and that concern for the worst off is triggering effective and widely spun improvements.

Since a view from nowhere is inconceivable, so a non-fictional work is bound to the fictional way the world is viewed by reason, science and observation delivering "objective" versions inevitably sifted and shaped by social contexts. Kant believed that reality in itself *–das Ding an sich–* could never be grasped, but this is an antinomy: how to know that the ungraspable exists? In numerous variations, Horkheimer and Adorno's *Dialects of Enlightenment* (1947) disavowed any discipline's claim to pursue knowledge and truth in an objective way free from contextual influence: "As solid citizens, philosophers ally themselves in practice with the powers they condemn in theory."

The idea of writing about diseased people, who for a diversity of causes do not receive medical and public health attention available in societies armed with resources and social policies that are comprehensive enough to secure healthcare equity, is far from being the straightforward enterprise that a first approach might suggest.

There is something pathetic in the insistence that humane healthcare should need bioethics as a reminder of the virtues that medicine and public healthcare ought to have engraved in their innermost core of practice, especially since bioethics has in many aspects not done its job. In fact, bioethics has dodged any obligation to look deeply into the dark crevices of neglected populations unable to access the benefits of basic medical and public healthcare to treat what the World Health Organization calls "preventable diseases". Time and again, bioethics is conceived as centered on clinical ethics and biomedical research ethics, at best amplifying their scope to address concerns about resources allocation in scarcity, and condescending to throw brief glances at ecological issues.

There are, of course, exceptions, and this book pretends to be one. Hopefully, it cannot be classified: the text is not scholarly enough to satisfy academia, nor is it sufficiently unburdened to be introductory or popularizing. Inevitably, a longer than preferable list of references has accumulated to sustain or reject certain empirical assertions, dissect matters of importance from matters of fact, as Whitehead suggested, and nudge bioethics to take some unusual directions. Little of what is said has not been presented before and, like any blend or medley, it is not the components but the mix that pretends some originality.

The book, should it reach more than a handful of readers, will irritate by its iconoclastic views on some untouchable concepts like human rights, dignity, solidarity, global ethics, and more. It has an undeniable tendency towards profanation as understood by Giorgio Agamben: "Profane –writes the great jurist Trebatius– properly refers to that which having been sacred or religious, is returned to the use and ownership of men."

Criticism without desacralizing some deeply entrenched current discourses offers little hope of deflating exuberant proclamations promising to solve the issue of healthcare in Low Income Countries (LIC) by 2045, all the more discouraging when relying on economic assistance and technical innovation which, being much of the same, have had hardly any substantial effect on structures of power and the reduction of inequality.

> In the absence of major medical advances, CMNN [communicable, maternal, neonatal and nutritional health disorders] causes are likely to remain dominant health challenges among the poorest countries, and there is a real risk that the HIV epidemic could rebound in many countries if progress is not maintained. Continued technical innovation and heightened spending on health, inclusive of development assistance for health, will be necessary to prevent millions of people from living in substantially worse conditions than the rest of the world. (Foreman et al. 2018)

*Introduction*                                                    xiii

Taking neglected diseases as a prime example of healthcare inequity requires a guarded and critical view of some deeply accepted values like progress, the conquests of scientific knowledge and technical know-how, and a generalized tendency towards equating well-being with an insatiable consumption of modern life's commodities. The shadows cast by this luminous and uplifting scenario become distant and alien, blurring and masking an immense number of human beings living in the negativities of unmet basic needs, endlessly toiling to escape from absolute poverty and endure the relative poverty of bare subsistence, cringing under the burdens of unattended, life-shortening disease, and the relentless heredity of misfortune.

Should we care?

This book is presented in the conviction that human beings should care for humanity and humaneness.

*Chapter 1*

# RIGHTS AND JUSTICE

## I. HUMAN RIGHTS

Thomas Jefferson penned the Declaration of Independence (1776) declaring, for the first time that "All men are created equal…endowed by their Creator with certain unalienable Rights, that among these are Life, Liberty and the Pursuit of Happiness." The immediate response of abolitionist Thomas Day was: "If there be an object truly ridiculous in nature, it is an American patriot, signing resolutions of independency with the one hand, and with the other brandishing a whip over his affrighted slaves."

According to Article 1 of the French Declaration of the Rights of Man and of the Citizen (1789), "Men are born and remain free and equal in rights. Social distinctions may be founded only upon the general good." And yet, ink was mixed with blood during the 1793-94 Reign of Terror, where the feminist writer Olympe de Gouges, having published in 1791 the Declaration of the Rights of Woman and the Female Citizen, was among those guillotined for treason. In 1948, at the end of worldwide atrocities perpetrated during the first half of the century, the Universal Declaration of Human Rights was proclaimed (1948), headed by article 1: "All human beings are born free and equal in dignity and rights... ." The same year, Richard M. Weaver published his book *Ideas Have Consequences* stating that, "no man was ever created free and no two men ever created equal." If equality were ever to be achieved, it would not be on the basis of a "chimerical notion of equality but upon fraternity."

Familial and educational influences are primarily instrumental in constructing the socially adapted uniqueness of each person so that, *de facto*, the statement that human beings are born free and equal in dignity and rights is a hollow assertion in the face of social and political aims at creating a social composite of undifferentiated monads, unequal in status, role, opportunities and contexts, yet supposed to enjoy equality in rights and duties. Human rights are often used as underpinnings of current ethical thought ignoring the vagaries and inconsistencies that the vaguely defined discourse on human rights has been subject to.

Prepared and proclaimed in the aftermath of World War II, the Universal Declaration of Human Rights (UDHR) was a reactive document stressing the need to respect and under no circumstances violate the human rights to life, liberty, security, and recognition "everywhere as a person before the law". These first-generation or negative rights proscribed maleficence in the form of torture, slavery or "degrading treatment or punishment". Although a general formulation of positive rights was presented, the Declaration has been mainly concerned with denouncing the violation of basic rights by rogue states. Though constantly invoked, the UDHR has little power beyond shaming and blaming, a role coherently exercised and widely respected, though with scant corrective power.

> The real trouble about human rights, when historically correlated with market fundamentalism, is not that they promote it but that they are unambitious in theory and ineffectual in practice in the face of market fundamentalism's success.
>
> The tragedy of human rights is that they have occupied the global imagination but have so far contributed little of note, merely nipping at the heels of the neoliberal giant whose path goes unaltered and unresisted. (Moyn 2018, 4435)

It took almost two decades to elaborate the twin Covenants that specifically proclaimed universal economic, social and cultural rights, in

*Rights and Justice* 3

addition to civil and political rights, and another half century to conclude that

> Material subversion of socio-economic rights, the era of neo-liberal globalization –with its emphasis on commodification, commercialization and privatization– fundamentally undermines the enjoyment of basic socio-economic rights for millions of people around the world. (O'Connell 2011, 534)

The U.N. considers covenants to be legally binding for signatory States, yet necessarily tempers compliance by contextualizing their realization, and by setting goals at an unrealistic level. The International Covenant on Economic, Social and Cultural Rights (1966) is unambiguous about national obligations to progressively comply within their available means.

> Part II. Art. 2. Each State Party to the present Covenant undertakes to take steps, individually and through international assistance and co-operation, especially economic and technical, to the maximum of its available resources, with a view to achieving progressively the full realization of the rights recognized in the present Covenant by all appropriate means, including particularly the adoption of legislative measures.

As for goals, rights are presented in such an undetermined form that they cannot be claimed by "everyone", nor can the States be made accountable for failing to comply with the "right of everyone to an adequate standard of living for himself and his family." Perhaps the most abstruse reference to healthcare matters is the ethereally formulated "right of everyone to the enjoyment of the highest attainable standard of physical and mental health." Understandably, such hyperbolic language elicits negative comments such as

The Declaration defines rights poorly, and says almost nothing about the corresponding duties. No inspection of the *Universal Declaration*, or of later UN or European documents, shows *who* is required to do *what*, or *why* they are required to do it. The underlying difficulty of any declaration of rights is that it assumes a *passive* view of human life and of citizenship. (O'Neill 2002, 28)

Taking into consideration the sixty years that separate us from the 1948 Declaration, it becomes impossible to state that fundamental rights extend to all human beings, or even that there has been a significant reduction in the number of those who do not have a satisfactory guarantee of their vital needs being covered. Despite abundant rhetoric about humanitarian commitments, human life continues to be to a great degree excluded from lawful protection, to the point that it becomes difficult to affirm that, even in the frame of increasing juridification of society, no right has been so neglected as the life of millions of human beings condemned to certain death by hunger, disease, war. (Esposito 2009, 110)

Human rights, focused on securing enough for everyone, are essential –but they are not enough. (Moyn 2018, xii)

Recent scholarly work has unveiled evidence that the "1950 European Convention on Human Rights" was "an individualistic and conservative project...designed to stem the postwar tide of socialism and statism" (Stephen Sedley in the London Review of Books 30 August 2018). Such criticism can surely be extended to the UDHR.

The rights historian Samuel Moyn discusses how human rights discourse has wavered between its call for national welfare states, and the later emergence of a quest for global justice.

But with human rights in ethics and neoliberalism in economics arising, with the national welfare state in crisis and with initial visions of a more ambitious globalized welfare nipped in the bud, the ideal of equality died. The idea of sufficiency was left to subside alone. (Moyn 2018, 117)

## Rights and Justice

Or, as often pointed out, universality is claimed even though reality ignores it. Even merging both views, as some scholars have suggested, neglected populations fail to be included, mainly because ever since the seminal work of Thomas Marshall, rights refer to citizenship. Marginalized and neglected populations fall under the category of human beings who do not have "the right to have rights" as Hannah Arendt says. The stateless, the migrants, and the marginalized poor have no standing on which to claim any rights at all, and any concept of human rights simply does not reach them. Human beings who are denied the right to have rights, belong to what Bauman calls the "underclass":

> The meaning of the 'underclass identity' is an *absence of identity*; the effacement or denial of individuality, of 'face' –that object of ethical duty and moral care. You are cast outside the social space in which identities are sought, chosen, constructed, evaluated, confirmed, or refuted. (Bauman 2005, 39)

Agamben refers to human beings whose *bios* –human life as socially and politically integrated– has been demoted to the state of *zoe* –purely animal life–, as an occurrence in states of exceptionality, pointing out that "exceptionality" has become regularly incorporated into contemporaneous democracies. From an anthropological view, human beings stripped down to animality cannot survive, for they lack the instinctual equipment to directly cover their vital necessities, described by Primo Levi as the *Muselmänner*, their imminent death written on their face, the "non-men", hardly to be considered living.

> To recall Thomas Marshall's famous triad of rights: economic rights are now out of the state's hands, such political rights as states may offer are strictly limited and kept inside of what Pierre Bourdieu baptised as *pensée unique* of the thoroughly deregulated free market neoliberal style, while social rights are replaced one by one by the individual duty of self-care and one-upmanship. (Bauman 2005, 28)

6                                Miguel Kottow

Can the UDHR be invoked even though it is clearly not universal, and in spite of having been heavily criticized, and unheeded in reality? Has the Declaration had any practical effect on world affairs, in the wake of increasing socioeconomic disparities, stagnant statistics on malnutrition, and famine? Can phrases like "right to health" or "right to healthcare" be disambiguated in a meaningful way and captured to secure a correlative duty of performance?

Quite a few theorists have shown that accounts of rights face the constant dilemma between being either universal and abstract or local and concrete. Furthermore, the distinction between negative and positive, just as the separation between rights and duties, promotes misunderstandings rather than enlightenment.

> One declares a *right* to be left alone as a means of appealing to some third parties for protection against those second parties who will in fact not choose to leave others alone. If even this meager appeal for protection against violators is to be granted, then, besides a duty to leave others alone that must fall upon everyone –a universal duty of non-interference– a duty to protect right-bearers against second-parties who violate their universal duty of non-interference must fall upon at least some third parties. (Shue 2004, 224)

The meaning of human rights differs in different cultures, Asian thought having criticized their individualistic slant that fails to understand the trans-individual connections with ancestry, family and nature.

As in all its documents and proclamations, the CESCR is an agreement between most member states, necessarily resorting to a bland language that acknowledges that national resource constraints may set the pace to act as best they can within their means. Every nation will have to contextualize the fulfillment of basic positive human rights, like healthcare, facing the reality that

> Institutional human rights are not, strictly speaking, unmodified *human* rights. They will, rather, bear much resemblance to *political* rights, which are recognized by particular states on the basis of their own

*Rights and Justice*                                                7

particular political culture and value priorities. (Arras and Fenton 2009, 35)

This is a conclusion that the authors had anticipated when stating that "a right to health-related goods is compatible with the unfortunate likelihood that it will not be honored for the majority of the world's poor for many years to come" (Ibid. 32).

No global actions are put on the table, no suggestions of international assistance or subsidiary economic aid can be read into the doctrine of national progressive realization, failing to explicitly acknowledge how socioeconomic factors are the principal determinants in the dire consequences of worldwide inequity. What is ignored remains neglected.

## II. THE UNIVERSAL DECLARATION OF BIOETHICS AND HUMAN RIGHTS (UNBHR)

The United Nations Educational, Scientific and Cultural Organization (UNESCO) devoted two years of deliberations to prepare and proclaim the UNBHR in 2005, considered "as an important step in the search for global bioethical standards...Its main goal is...to assemble some basic standards to help states in their efforts to promote responsible biomedical research and clinical practice, in conformity with the principles of international human rights law" (Andorno 2007, 153). The Declaration has received mixed reviews, hailed as a milestone but also criticized, among other things, for its Western principlist perspective based on dignity and human rights considered by many to be the product of European enlightenment philosophy.

It does seem odd that the United Nations should have deemed it necessary to formally connect human rights with bioethics at such a late date, given that it is obvious that any form of ethics, and certainly bioethics, is transcendentally anchored in human rights, that is, confirming that the necessary condition of any ethics is the acceptance of basic human rights, however they are defined. Although this intrinsic link between bioethics and human rights is weak and unstable, it certainly will not become more robust because UNESCO says so: "Human dignity, human rights and fundamental freedoms are to be fully respected" (Article 3(1)). This tripod of concepts is far too precarious to serve as groundwork for such an ambitious proclamation.

The Declaration avoids mentioning neglected diseases or orphan maladies, preferring to "recognize the importance of freedom of scientific research and the benefits derived from scientific and technological developments" (Art. 2(d)). Who is to benefit if the pharmaceutical industry prefers to search for a blockbuster drug instead of directing R&D to unprofitable vaccines or to orphan drugs, which are only lucrative if highly priced? Freedom of research exempts science from any social responsibility to explore palliative or therapeutic ways of helping the destitute and marginalized needy, flying in the face of Art. 15(b) of the International Covenant on Economic, Social and Cultural Rights: "The States Parties to the present Covenant recognize the right of everyone to enjoy the benefits of scientific progress and its applications."

A major inconsistency of the UDBHR is its blatant assertion that "This Declaration is addressed to States" (Art. 1, 2), and yet, it has universal aspirations that pretend to go well beyond national sovereignty and jurisdiction. The first of its "Aims" is "to provide a universal framework of principles and procedures to guide States in the formulation of their legislation, policies or other instruments in the field of bioethics." Utterly and perhaps purposefully confusing.

## III. SOCIOECONOMIC "DETERMINANTS"

The association of poverty and disease, mainly via faulty public hygiene, had long been known and was, in fact, the origin of public health in the 18th century, when J. P. Frank published his "*Medizinpolizei*". T. McKeown's classic work on the reduction of disease when material standards of living improved, and the statistical demonstration that diseases like tuberculosis dramatically decreased their prevalence long before vaccination and anti-tuberculosis medication were developed, convincingly relate socioeconomic development with better health, just as poverty is linked with disease.

Recognition of the worldwide prevalence of socioeconomic inequities that are worsened and cemented by globalization, has led to seeing these disparities as determinants, which is a roundabout way of acknowledging that the situation has also been naturalized and firmly anchored in the *status quo* of neoliberal globalization. If corrective global efforts were to be seriously implemented, a less pessimistic approach would refer to socioeconomic conditions, for a condition is more amenable to change than a determinant.

The social determinants of health are described by the WHO (Social Determinants of Health: Key Concepts), as "the circumstances in which people are born, grow up, live, work and age, and the systems put in place to deal with illness. These circumstances are in turn shaped by a wider set of forces: economics, social policies, and politics." The social determinants of health are largely responsible for health inequities within and between countries. Health, illness, disease and disability are outcomes of a number of social, cultural and economic factors that operate and interact at both the individual and population levels. These include income, housing, food security, early childhood development, education, healthcare, employment, the social and physical environment, culture, health behaviors, genetics and gender.

Socioeconomic determinants (SEDs) of global inequity have become increasingly troublesome since globalization has made disparity more acute, even though there is a torpid but encouraging reduction of world absolute poverty. The development charity Oxfam issued an update at the beginning of 2018: 42 people hold as much wealth as 3.7 billion of the poorest half of the world. The rich/poor gap widens literally by the day: 82% of the global wealth generated in 2017 went to the extremely wealthy 1%.

About 10.7% of the world population live on less than $1.90 per day, totaling about 750 million human beings who live in extreme poverty, unable to cover their basic biological needs. Statistics are elaborated by the

# 10                                 *Miguel Kottow*

World Bank using hard data where available, and extrapolations in less accessible, that is more destitute, areas.

Taking the $1.90 daily income –updated to $2.00– as a threshold of extreme poverty, statistics agree that there has been some improvement for millions of people that have crossed this parameter, provided it refers to absolute income poverty, without addressing relative poverty –relative deprivation and social exclusion–. In fact, mastering the income threshold decreases the prevalence of absolute poverty but increases the number of people living in underprivileged and precarious healthcare conditions.

Global inequality now presents as an elephant curve developed by economist Branko Milanovic showing how world poverty has decreased (elephant's high back), the middle classes' income has stagnated and relatively declined (elephant's lowered face), while the top earners are doing well (elevated and upward looking trunk) (Lanchester 2018). Global inequality is on the rise and, though the global Gini index has declined by two points to around 70.5 –still a high figure–, this apparent improvement probably is the artificial gain of under-reported top incomes (Lackner and Milanovic 2013).

The United Nations proclaimed the Millennium Development Goals (MDGs) in the year 2000, anticipating that poverty, hunger, disease, unmet schooling needs, gender inequality, and environmental degradation would be substantially decreased by 2015. Statistics confirmed notable progress due to major efforts in China and India, but the program was less successful in meeting the needs of the most underprivileged:

> The probable shortfall in achievement of the MDGs is indeed serious, regrettable, and deeply painful for people with low income. The shortfall represents a set of operational failures that implicate many stakeholders, in both poor and rich countries. Promises of official development assistance by rich countries, for example, have not been kept. (Sachs 2012, 2206)

An additional program known as Sustainable Development Goals (SDG) was presented to unfold actions focused on a combination of economic development, environmental sustainability, and social inclusion.

## Rights and Justice

> The SDGs will therefore need the unprecedented mobilisation of global knowledge operating across many sectors and regions. Governments, international institutions, private business, academia, and civil society will need to work together to identify the critical pathways to success, in ways that combine technical expertise and democratic representation. Global problem-solving networks for sustainable development –in energy, food, urbanisation, climate resilience, and other sectors– will therefore become crucial new institutions in the years ahead. (Ibid.)

Quoted is the highly praised and prized American economist Jeffrey D. Sachs who has actively worked in the above-mentioned U.N. programs, sharing caution and the satisfaction of goals reached, as well as the optimism of major success within the next two decades. Nevertheless, critics have claimed that poor countries are stuck in a "poverty trap" – Easterly–, and pointed out that Sachs' projects, though well intended, have "left people even worse off than before –Munk–, centering on assistance rather than empowerment that has "created dependence" –Theroux–. The undiminished negative forces of socioeconomic determinants, and the increasing market-induced economic polarization give reason to doubt that progress in favor of the poor is being achieved in a decisive way.

The OECD/DAC –Development Assistance Committee– introduced specific recommendations to raise external aid –Official Development Aid (ODA) to 0.7% of richer countries, mainly the European Union's Gross National Income, presented as the ODA/GNI target. Not all OECD countries signed this agreement, nor did most of the signatories honor it, so these well-meant efforts were uneven and with a tendency to decrease when world finances destabilized.

The current worldwide situation statistically confirms that socioeconomic gaps are on the rise, that the artificially set poverty line has been surpassed in many societies by slight increases in average income, and that some indicators show that hunger is down to a stable 800 million; a similar number of people lack basic drinking water sources globally, while at least 2 billion people use drinking water sources contaminated with feces. These and many additional statistics presented by the WHO, are actively juggled and disaggregated in order to support a variety of politically and ideologically inspired rhetoric.

Apart from being prone to error due to diversely reliable data sources, statistics may initially increase awareness of the magnitude of problems, but their endless repetition has an anaesthetizing effect. Susan Sontag's insightful work on war photography and the perception of the distant "pain of others", apply in full to the quantitative presentation of worldwide misery.

> To designate a hell is not, of course, to tell us anything about how to extract people from that hell, how to moderate hell's flames. Still, it seems a good in itself to acknowledge, to have enlarged, one's sense of how much suffering caused by human wickedness there is in the world we share with others. Someone who is perennially surprised that depravity exists, who continues to feel disillusioned (even incredulous) when confronted with evidence of what humans are capable of inflicting in the way of gruesome, hands-on cruelties upon other human beings, has not reached moral or psychological adulthood.
>
> No one after a certain age has the right to this kind of innocence, of superficiality, to this degree of ignorance or amnesia. (Sontag 2003, 114)

The massive numbers of distant suffering breed insensitivity with a tendency to naturalize socioeconomic disparities, and register them as a fact of life. Witnessed under any ethical lens, SEDs constitute a major injustice that needs to be redressed, going through such basic concepts as justice, distribution, sustainability, social minimum, humanitarian aid and solidarity, and gauging their conceptual pertinence to broach the problems of induced suffering and ignored remedies.

Sheer numbers, though impressive, lose impact through repetition, but the more transcendent message is the accelerated trend towards increased inequalities and their dire consequences. Anthropological fieldwork in India has demonstrated that "the coverage figures of immunization, as for other target-driven programs, tend to be upwardly biased by the hierarchical nature of record keeping in which targets and goals move from top to bottom while information moves from bottom to top" (Das 1999,

*Rights and Justice* 13

107-108). The injudicious use of antibiotics and persistent obstacles to completing vaccination programs favor the resistance of microorganisms and vectors that continue to thrive in poverty-stricken environments and trigger the re-emergence of previously controlled diseases, notably multidrug-resistant tuberculosis (MDR TB) and the still more unmanageable extensive drug-resistant TB (XDR TB).

Nor will numbers mask that socioeconomic disparities are dooming one-third of the world population to live on less than two dollars a day, condemning these human beings to an insufficient nutritional uptake, a lack of medical care and efficient public health, education and the minimal empowerment necessary to survive.

Leading English epidemiologist Sir Michael Marmot has written extensively on the subject he prefers to call "social inequalities". His influential work has emphasized the urgency of reaching health equity by identifying and correcting a series of major structural problems. Excerpts from his most recent publication are characteristic of the extensive knowledge and vague hope of improvement that feature in most studies on socioeconomic disparities and their negative consequences on the health, protection and minimal well-being of a vast majority of the human population:

> Health is a worthwhile goal for individuals and for communities… Better health and greater health equity will come when life chances and human potential are freed to create the conditions for all people to achieve their highest attainable standard of health and to lead dignified lives… . Reducing health inequities will remain elusive unless the structural drivers are addressed… . Structural drivers – e.g., large and growing economic inequalities, privileging of the private sector over recognition of the importance of a flourishing public domain, and ignoring the environment– must all be tackled in the pursuit of health equity. Our recommendations do not proceed on the assumption that addressing these structural drivers is easy. But health inequities provide powerful reasons for doing so. (Marmot 2018, 1, 2)

SEDs pretend to be a descriptive issue that eases the way to some kind of normative global perspectives, notably aiming at global health. The most pertinent and effective global health venture is the contention and therapeutic advances in the HIV epidemic, hailed as a model for future worldwide healthcare ventures, a view that does not resist further analysis. The combined efforts of public health, medicine and biomedical research have been effective in reducing the incidence of, and halving death rates due to HIV/AIDS, but underlying SEDs remain of unmitigated importance, as confirmed by the fact that poverty-ridden sub-Saharan populations in Africa continue to have the highest prevalence rates of HIV infection. Another atypical feature is that concern over the HIV pandemic was triggered by its sudden spread in prosperous Western nations. Single diseases, least of all HIV/AIDS can hardly be paradigmatic for global health programs:

> Global is not merely a constellation of diseases, a collection of national health systems, or even a set of values. It is a way of looking at our world. It seeks to observe, document, monitor, interpret and eliminate the harms that accrue from national and transnational forces inimical to health –political, commercial, military, financial, diplomatic, legal, intersectional, and cultural. Global health is about power and poverty, violence and exploitation, oppression and silence, and collusion and exclusion. (Horton 2018)

Holistic views may be inspiring, but they have unrealistic views with little bite and credibility as shown by a WHO/TDR report understanding that its mandate is to "strengthen the capacity of developing endemic countries to undertake the research required for developing and implementing these new and improved disease control approaches" (Hunt 2007, 3). As often seen, this is a case of "think global" –a holistic view of health problems– "act local" –national implementation–. The scenario of health threatening problems triggered by modern lifestyles includes travel, migrations, trade and international markets, the urbanization of animals, facilitated transmission of vectors and infectious agents, eventually leading to rapidly spreading pandemics –$H_1N_1$, SARS–. Global health problems are

*Rights and Justice* 15

impervious to unfocused global healthcare measures that prove unable to manage the contagiousness of modern lifestyle changes.

## IV. GLOBALIZATION AND GLOBAL ETHICS

The nice way of seeing globalization is as a primarily economic process of worldwide integration and expanding consumer-based well-being, studded with terms like human flourishing and happiness. A more critical and realistic view shows deep rifts between the powerful minority that benefits, and the severe negative consequences suffered by vast segments of the world's population. Globalization, originally of national scope, has become an international economic process strongly influencing the production and marketing of goods and services, the expansive flow of information in growing cyberspace, causing *"the outbreak of politics* from the framework of the national State, furthermore affecting the role structure *–Rollenschematik* – of what is considered 'political' or 'nonpolitical' action" (Beck 1998, 13). Globalization has been developing for some time, expanding and trailing "its associated litany of problems – uneven development, monocultural blandness, environmental degradation, anti-Western resentment" (Kidd 2005, 14).

Hans Tietmeyer, onetime president of Germany's Federal Bank, presented some of the necessary conditions to encourage investments. To gain the trust of investors and incite them to invest, he said, a more strict control of public expenditure is required, as well as tax reforms restructuring the system of social protection, and efforts to "to dismantle the labor market's rigidities" (Bauman 2001, 136).

Globalized institutions like international banks –the World Bank, the International Monetary Fund– sign treaties that reduce national sovereignty over laws concerning labor, healthcare, social security, tax systems, and educational policies, facilitate foreign investment and usurp national governance. National political action is displaced or replaced by the neoliberal ideology of global market dominance. Globalization has reduced and transformed the role of the national State (Mamdani 2018).

16                                 *Miguel Kottow*

> The neglect of these problems [world health] is everywhere. Foreign aid is minimal, despite some posturing and promising. Research done by drug companies is largely directed at new drugs for chronic diseases of those who can pay, which do not include most of the world's poor. Agricultural research, which might help alleviate malnutrition, is also minimally concerned with the problems of food production in the poorest countries. Research funding from governments of rich countries is also largely designed to help with problems faced by the citizens of those countries. (Baron 2006, 206)

Global ethics presupposes the reawakening of solidarity, and the widespread establishment of a democratic, grassroots "cosmopolitan parliament" (Fraser) to develop ethical policies and decision-making processes, by activating deliberative democracy –Habermas– or reflexive equilibrium –Rawls– especially to resolve bioethical issues –Daniels–. Such holistic proposals are at odds with reality, giving more and more credence to Rorty's resignation at the repeated mistake of holding reality and justice in a single vision.

Beyond good intentions, there are strong reasons to doubt that any form of global tendency to reduce inequality might be on its way; well-rounded proclamations are at best anesthetizing the urgent need to broach distal roots of inequity, while failing to remedy proximal sources of harm.

Sociologist Hauke Brunkhorst has perceptively analyzed the legitimation of social and institutional forces of inclusion/exclusion policies and their impact on inequalities. Democracies are pledged to the universal goal of *"exclusion of inequalities"*, as pursued by the "nation state" empowered to *"exclude inequalities* with respect to *individual rights, political participation* and *equal access to social welfare and opportunities."* Universalistic ambitions of human rights declarations, and pervading political and economic globalization have contributed to the "decay of the ability of the nation state to exclude inequalities", explaining why the *"national exclusion of inequality* no longer is successful". Solidarity breaks up as a *"new rule"* of the *"cosmopolitism of the few* (Calhoun) emerges", hindering that global politics universally be committed to the *"exclusion of inequalities"* (Brunkhorst, undated). Rather, as some inequalities are excluded, new inequalities are included, bringing to mind Michel Foucault's concept of biopolitics: the traditional pre-modern right of sovereignty was to let live by making die, in other words, to defend the survival of sovereignty by eliminating its enemies. Modern biopower adds the right to make live and let die that is, prosperous living for some means letting others shrivel and die because of unfulfilled basic needs.

Global ethicists try to ignore that neoliberal globalization has become the only viable political strategy after socialism crumbled or negotiated its entrance into market economies. There are potent reasons to admit the irreversibility of this trend and its resilience when suffering economic backlashes that seem to weaken the system's foundations but finally allow it to resurface unscathed and even strengthened. According to economist Vito Tanzi, the expansion of globalization will include strategies that will decrease national tax revenues, thus exacerbating social and international inequality, deepening the plight of the underprivileged.

A fundamental ethical worldview would strive for universally fair social conditions and equal moral treatment throughout everyone's existence, including care and protection for the weak, educational opportunities for the growing, job openings for active adults, and secure pensions and social integration for the elderly. Such a view requires concern for a common weal robust enough at the national level to deliver fair treatment to all. National prosperity in today's world is unachievable unless mutually supportive international trade agreements and policies are sought, a requirement that is unthinkable in a climate of global competitiveness with predominant neoliberal politics and economics evolving at the cost of mounting inequalities and weakening national resources and social responsibilities.

## V. SUSTAINABILITY AND DISTRIBUTION

The idea of sustainable development was first presented by the United Nation's Brundtland Commission (1987) as: "development that meets the needs of the present without compromising the ability of future generations to meet their own needs." Caring about future generations had been one of the main themes of Hans Jonas' *The Imperative of Responsibility* (1984), requesting that technoscientific expansion reverts to a "frugal" and precautionary pace in view of the incommensurable negative consequences that would otherwise ensue for the present and future survival of mankind.

A widely used concept, sustainability requires moderation in the use of natural resources and care to reduce pollution, yet obscures the fact that resources ought only to be reduced if they are sufficient to cover the needs of all actual populations. It is unreasonable and unethical to save resources for the future when one-third of humanity lacks essential goods like water, nutrition, medication, shelter and basic security. Under these conditions, the costs of sustainability for future generations burden the now poor and deprived. The question arises whether sustainability should consider not only the production of resources, but also their distribution, considering that wealthy nations' consumption for most types of primary energy resources exceeds by far the availability for poor regions, let alone the poorest population in disadvantaged areas. Sustainable development – exploiting natural resources, producing and consuming goods– can only be gauged once it is assured that energy production does in fact meet the basic needs of the world population, and allows a remnant to be saved for the future.

Protecting the needs of future generations remains an unknown since there is no way of anticipating the quantity and quality of future needs. Saving for the future is mandatory provided the needs of the present have been met, developing policies that not only regulate production but also cap overconsumption of goods and services exercised by middle- and high-income countries. John Locke would say that sustainability is reasonable "at least where there is enough, and as good, left in common for others", that is, distribution schemes are acceptable provided no one suffers want.

Rights and Justice 19

# VI. Distributive Justice

When Jon Elster writes that "the cart of procedural justice ought not to be put before the horse of substantive justice" (Miller 1999, 105), he means that distributive justice becomes a live concept if it says something about *what* is to be distributed and to *whom*. The classical definition of justice requires citizens to live honestly, hurt no one, give everyone his due. It revives the Aristotelian idea of justice as an absolute virtue of the individual. In modernity dominated by reason and the subservience of values and virtues to an economic language of achievements, the idea of fleshing out some form of social justice is frustrating and fruitless. It becomes much simpler to describe situations of injustice, like poverty or unfair treatment, and leave it at that without further engagement, somehow blending with the traditional and romantic idea that being poor is no disgrace for they are blessed, as expressed by Leo XIII in *Auspicato concessum* (1882):

> ...the question that politicians so laboriously aim at solving, viz., the relations which exist between the rich and the poor, would be thoroughly solved if they held this as a fixed principle, viz., that poverty is not wanting in dignity; that the rich should be merciful and munificent, and the poor content with their lot and labour; and since neither was born for these changeable goods, the one is to attain heaven by patience the other by liberality. (Schuck 1991, 82)

While it would be politically incorrect and morally unsound to approve this Papal view, it still lies dormant but not extinguished in many diverse stances taken to discourage human beings from tampering with "natural" processes by "playing God". A nudge towards justice is expressed in *Populorum progression* (Paul VI, 1967): "No one is justified in keeping for his exclusive use what he does not need, when others lack necessities" (Ibid., 147). In the midst of the Cold War, distance from Marxism meant giving support to a friendly capitalism –a social market economy–. As neoliberal globalization reigns unrivaled, the quest for justice becomes more ethereal and polymorphic, as an extreme form of capitalism, often called "savage", sharpens its bullish horns.

The enormous academic production on social justice insistently asserts –perhaps with the exception of recalcitrant libertarians– that poverty is not a natural condition, but rather the product of the privileged taking advantage of the unfortunate. If poverty is man-made, so should its remedy be; consequently, efforts should not be orientated towards the utopia of justice, but to world affairs that are causing injustice. And yet, a vivid discussion has surfaced and is known as the "Equality of what" debate. Obvious common sense would dictate that the quest for abolishing injustice is to remove inequality –egalitarianism– by reforming the way goods and services are actually distributed, an unreachable goal since it would require taking from the wealthy to benefit the worse off, also an impossible dream given the firm grounding of a *status quo* that welds wealth to power.

The alternative to seeking justice by enforcing equality is to strive for social and economic conditions that will protect the poor from need and provide them with the empowerment to improve their lot. Egalitarianism is countered by a "doctrine of sufficiency".

> From the point of view of morality, it is not important that everyone should have the *same*. What is morally important is that each should have *enough*. If everyone had enough money, it would be of no special or deliberate concern whether some people had more money than others. (Frankfurt 2015, 7)

Certainly, Frankfurt is too prominent as a philosopher to believe that mentioning "*enough*" is enough, as he acknowledges that egalitarianism helps smooth the turbulences of a sufficiency doctrine, but quoting him eases the way towards recognizing that the worse off are better served by concern for a social minimum than insisting on unattainable equality. Swaying between egalitarianism and sufficiency has also been the mark of human rights doctrines, at present favoring sufficiency over the impassable contradiction of egalitarian globalization.

*Rights and Justice* 21

John Locke's idea of an initially equal distribution of natural resources, accepting that luck and hard work would in all fairness soon lead to tolerable inequality and the polarization of economic power, provided that "claiming ownership has no negative effect upon others". What is fairly owned, may be processed to increase its value, and profitably transferred to transactions in a market that operates within the moral limits of fairness, decency and autonomous actions. Luck and competence will play to the advantage of the industrious, creating an inequality gap where losers have no claim for redress, unless foul play requires rectification. In libertarian Robert Nozick's view, even though inequalities will be inherited throughout generations, Locke's proviso will continue to cast a "historical shadow" allowing equal opportunities to ensure the survival of all. But neoliberalism evolves in a way that unrelentingly dismantles the idea of equality at birth, and proclaims equal opportunities that do not obtain in an unequal world. "A community of emancipated men does not constitute a society. The idea of social equality is a contradiction *in adjecto*" as J. Rancière has written when pointing out that a community of equals becomes a society where diversified functions, roles and production breed inequality.

There are some unpalatable consequences that cannot be easily accounted for when considering that inequalities are passed on for generations as if they were some sort of hereditary genetic dominance. Secondly, past injustice may have been respectful of law and morals at the time they were committed, only much later decried and abolished with no retroactive compensatory considerations for harm done. Slavery was perfectly respectful when Aristotle wrote about the ethics of virtue, and the best modern states have disregarded their slave-mongering past and yet ignore the amending of harms and injuries for persistent discriminations. Legally sought reparations have been few and ill fated, setting a precedent that holds for past actions that were, but no longer are, morally and legally justified, although the consequences of these injuries continue to plague their descendants. Redress for past injustice has often been argued against colonialism, and is also part of Pogge's justification of a Health Investment

Fund (see Chapter 7, 5-B), but actual reparation by positive discrimination is obtained only rarely if at all.

## VII. Social Minimum

The right to sufficiency of basic needs is closely knit with the issue of a social minimum, defined as

> That bundle of resources which suffices in the circumstances of a given society to enable someone to lead a minimally decent life. We define a 'social minimum policy regime' as a set of policies and institutions that serve to secure reasonable access to this social minimum of all members of the society. (White 2015, 1)

White's review article takes pains to clarify the notion of a "minimal decent life", and the diversity of approaches that have been presented. "Welfarism" refers to happiness or, according to Sen, to capabilities that allow "functioning" in quest of satisfaction of "elementary things" to attain happiness, social integration, "and so on" (Ibid., 6). In her own version of capabilities, Martha Nussbaum lists three that are of a biological nature – survival, health, and integrity–, and seven markedly cultural capabilities including imagination, emotional response, and play. All these approaches –utilitarianism, libertarianism in its various forms, and democratic perspectives– remain highly controversial, failing to define poverty and the "bundle of resources necessary for someone to live a minimally decent life *"in their society"* (Ibid., 11). Questions about the legitimacy of policies favoring the social minimum are often presented, especially in regard to the meaning of a "decent life" and the arbitrary listing of capabilities.

The distinction between absolute and relative poverty can also pertinently be applied to the social minimum: in its absolute meaning it related to a survival minimum, whereas the relative social minimum would consider the context of *"their* society" in which a minimum of empowerment is necessary to pursue a person's life within her social environment.

A pertinent debate ensues when applying the "capability of bodily health" which ranks highly in Nussbaum's list, and the healthcare needed to secure the social minimum by exercising relevant capabilities. The pertinent decision-making process ought to include: publicity, reasonableness, contestability, and enforcement (Daniels and Sabin 1997). Thus, the legitimacy of healthcare provision under a social minimum policy would be ensured.

White's article on the social minimum ends with the mention of issues that were not approached despite their importance: "If the government provides citizens with assistance in meeting a specific need, should it provide assistance in the form on 'in-kind' benefits or in the form of cash?" (White 2015, 52).

This question can only be asked from the perspective of high-income countries with a substantial corpus of prosperous scholars. It is unthinkable that poor individuals could satisfy their basic needs with income or cash assistance, considering that their buying-power depends on contextual realities like pricing, governmental subsidy, availability, accessibility, empowerment, and market negotiation that the poor may have had little opportunity to develop beyond bartered food transactions: "Secondly...What kind of obligations (if any) do we, as citizens of one country, have to secure the enactment of a social minimum in other countries?" (Ibid., 67). This is a major issue that is germane to the problems, debates and suggested solutions relating to the reality of neglected populations that will recur as the focus is sharpened on these matters.

## VIII. REDISTRIBUTION

Distribution is essentially a descriptive account of the whereabouts of certain goods in short supply. Original access to plentiful goods becomes a moral issue when availability is threatened by man-made interventions that create inequities in access gravitating in favor of some and scarcity for others. Accumulative distribution is not an innocent advantage gained by luck and hard work, as Locke suggested, but rather an exercise in power aimed at appropriation that leaves victims in a state of underprivileged vulnerability and susceptible to harm and decline.

Manipulation of, and intervention in, natural processes together with marked population growth, accelerate the misdistribution of every imaginable good –productive land, clean air, unpolluted water, care of the body, physical protection and social integration– polarize humanity between the powerful and plentiful, and the marginalized needy, with an intermediate great mass of strugglers fending to "make a living" and expending efforts at being productive and accepted members of a consumer society. This state of affairs results in inequality and the distressing awareness that economic values have become dominant and omnivorous, and that distribution inequities create harm and resentment, nourishing and often inflaming claims for distributive justice.

The woes of misdistribution call for redistribution, well captured by the German term *Umverteilung* suggesting change rather than mere adaptation. Libertarians and adherents of neoliberalism are insensitive to any problem of distribution by believing in a universal equality of opportunities that will sift winners from losers in a race without handicaps, no holds barred and freed from superior regulation beyond some rules that assure an undisturbed market system functioning with a lubricated offer/demand rhythm. This is a perhaps a too cynical description of contemporary socioeconomic goings on, but despite contextual overlays that hide the sheer harshness of contemporary life, the stark reality is that distribution is replaced by accumulation. The toxic and lethal effects are caused by overheated economies often decried by ecologists and defenders of sustainable growth yet denied by technophiles convinced that science and technology's benefits will neutralize mistakes and harms.

In a first approach, misdistribution is blamed on historical abuses of imperial domination, colonialism, ethnic discrimination, the reduction of women to the unfree private sphere of family life, and the marginalization of outsiders, ethnic minorities, and the weak. The argument that past

*Rights and Justice* 25

situations should be evaluated in their historic context is double-edged. Moral values are embedded in time and place and should be judged accordingly and, therefore, it is argued that historical periods of imperialist forms of colonialism, maltreatment, even enslavement, have come to an end, and should not be blamed for the present poverty and underdevelopment of former colonies. Contrariwise, it is plausibly argued that certain acts and policies enforced in the past have caused irreversible and ongoing damage that should be relieved, redressed, and cleansed by supportive trade and assistance agreements.

Arguably, distributive justice is the nuclear issue that concerns modern secular ethical thought, though the idea of justice has little purchase in the real world unless criteria for the distribution of goods and services are specified. As occurs with health, human rights, dignity, recognition and other rarified concepts are more visible in the negative forms of unhealthiness, violation of rights, offenses to dignity, misrecognition, and injustice.

The widely held impression that attempts to reassemble distribution through taxes is a liberal form of seeking fairness, criticized by socialist thinkers because the basic structure of capitalistic production remains untouched and will reproduce inequities that might have been temporarily reduced. Distribution may refer to resources, rights, accessibility to basic goods, government responsibilities, tax schemes, or constitutional legitimations. Equating generational distribution is much in the mind of societies concerned with the rapid increase of an unprotected elderly population.

Many proposals of redistribution are no more than flights of the imagination, more celebrated by their inventiveness than by expectations of feasibility. A more realistic approach addresses specific distributive distortions by proposing focal interventions –notably in healthcare issues– that promise symptomatic relief while acknowledging that structural obstacles will continue to work against permanent improvements.

Two main forms of facing injustice are redistribution and recognition, as exercised in the dialogic debate between Nancy Fraser and Axel Honneth that is germane to an ethical approach to neglect and injustice in healthcare. Although being theoretic propositions, they present frameworks that may be developed by practical reason and have, in fact, inspired social movements of recognition and redress for repressed majorities –feminism– and discriminated minorities –migrants and displaced groups, ethnic and racial communities–.

The quest for social justice is foremost in the work of both philosophers, acknowledging that two types of approach are currently predominant: 1) The claim for the redistribution of material goods and wealth between the poor and the rich, North and South and, in a somewhat outdated discourse, between capitalism and labor. The prevalence of the market economy has sidetracked retribution discourse into the theoretical realm; and 2) The upsurge of a politics and ethics of recognition inspired in the acknowledgement of differences –gender, culture, and ethnicity– in a world that should honor the equality of rights and just treatment. Redistribution and recognition must concur, with Fraser emphasizing the first, and Honneth the latter.

## A. Participatory Parity

The American philosopher Nancy Fraser's perspective develops from her strong commitment to feminism and advocacy for the *New Left,* acknowledging that claims for egalitarian redistribution have declined and given way to the politics of recognition. To her mind, social recognition drives many conflicts in different parts of the world to seek social justice by *participative parity.* Her emphasis on participation is a political call for equality in the social status of the many public spheres existing in a more complex contemporaneous society. The dichotomy between redistribution and recognition is false as she stresses that there can be no redistribution without recognition. Her understanding is that "status recognition" goes together with claims for equality: feminism needed to be acknowledged as a legitimate movement militating against gender inequality.

# Rights and Justice

Each dimension, moreover, is associated with an analytically distinct form of injustice. For the recognition dimension, as we saw, the associated injustice is misrecognition. For the distributive dimension, in contrast, the corresponding injustice is maldistribution, in which economic structures, property regimes or labour markets deprive actors of the resources needed to full participation. Each dimension, finally, corresponds to an analytically distinct form of subordination: the recognition dimension corresponds, as we saw, to status subordination, rooted in institutionalized patterns of cultural value; the distributive dimension, in contrast, corresponds to economic subordination, rooted in structural features of the economic system. (Fraser 2000, 6)

Fraser's thoughts apply to social groups struggling to assert their identity in order to gain equal participation in political *deliberation*. The active commitment refers to the emancipatory self-determination and self-assertion of individuals and groups, whereas political activism for status equality is a collective aim to be obtained in the political arena. Conscious that globalization is a strong opposing force to national or communal emancipation, Fraser believes that the public sphere ought to overcome the Westphalian concept of nation and strive towards a transnational democratic parliament. And yet, participative parity should be exercised not only in the political arena, but also in the realms of family, employment, the market, informal politics "as well as the various associations that are formed in civil society" (Ferrarese 2015). Fraser refers to "*ordinary-political misinterpretation*…which consists in the politically institutionalized denial of participatory parity among those who are already included in principle within a bounded polity" (Fraser 2009, 147).

Feminism has shown that "recognition respect," due equally to all human beings, does not reach secluded collectives subject to bias and discrimination by dominant groups that have historically disrespected women, ethnic minorities, distant majorities, and non-heterosexual communities. Retrieval of respect and equal recognition have been demanded through social mobilization and by the institution of a formal politics of recognition championing the causes of gender, race and ethnic diversities. Disempowerment of the aged and the loss of full recognition reduce them to so-called "second-groups". Marginalized, ignored, and neglected humans are noncitizens devoid of the recognition owed to their existence and basic rights. Fraser's status recognition is an unavailable instrument for neglected people who fail to have any presence in "bounded policies", lacking the necessary footing to embark on a struggle for recognition.

The status model of recognition takes issue with Honneth's theory of recognition as an inter-subjective aim at self-realization, and vice versa. "The war for social justice has therefore been short-changed into a plethora of battles for recognition" (Bauman 2005, 37).

## B. Recognition

Axel Honneth, Director of Frankfurt's famous Institute for Social Research, has centered his thoughts on social and interpersonal recognition as a quest for individual identity, the failure of which leads to injustice, discrimination and marginalization. In his view, social injustice is experienced when actual institutions operate with norms that individuals feel are damaging to their legitimate claims for social recognition. Taking a lead from Bourdieu's study on the miseries of the world showing that in most cases daily misery and suffering occur without reaching public awareness, Honneth works on the concept of intersubjective recognition in search of personal identity: "our notion of justice is also very closely linked to how, and as what, subjects mutually recognize each other" (Honneth 1997, 17). "Today, if we connect up with the concept of 'recognition' in order to introduce a concept of 'morality,' then the starting point is usually a phenomenological analysis of moral injuries" (Ibid., 22).

The idea that recognition is a fundamental part of human identity and moral worth was first elaborated by Hegel when describing the relationships and implicit norms derived from three spheres of recognition: love within the family, contractual respect within civil social structures, and solidarity within society at large (Iser 2013). Striving for identity and moral maturation by way of a multilayered process of recognition evolves

*Rights and Justice* 29

in an atmosphere of conflict and tension, characterized by Hegel as a struggle for recognition.

Based on Hegel's ideas on human ethical life –*Sittlichkeit*–, Honneth describes the three forms of moral support for recognition and identity formation: recognition of individual needs and desires supported by care and love provided by significant others –personal identity–; the recognition of moral accountability and equality in the treatment of moral respect – social interaction–; and recognition of a person's capability to be a valuable member of a concrete community, expressed in cooperation, solidarity or loyalty –moral obligation–.

Recognition is thus closely knitted with morality, in a negative way presenting levels of misrecognition as moral injuries. Injustice and moral harm relate to each one of these levels of self-relation: a) the moral injuries that rob a person's certainty of being able to enjoy physical well-being by harming bodily integrity through physical abuse; b) the moral injuries to capabilities of judgment and moral accountability, damaged by fraud, deceit or institutional discrimination; and c) the damage of humiliation caused when ignoring or denying that a person can be socially significant within a concrete community.

Both successful recognition and its distortion are socially mediated. All facets of self-identity need the acknowledgement of others, just as injuries to the self are produced by morally defective ways of denying recognition and respect to individuals or communities. Similar approaches refer to self-trust in choosing effectively, in acting competently, and in judging adequately.

Honneth's ethics of recognition addresses individual identity formation and social integration. Fraser, for her part, is concerned with the political recognition of communities seeking redress, justice and redistribution. Redistribution claims suggested by Fraser as participatory parity, presuppose that claimants are already grouped and struggling to eliminate discrimination and unequal treatment, as illustrated by the history of feminism, Gay Liberation, LGBT and similar movements. Patients, migrants, marginalized and neglected people are individuals hindered from having their moral rights recognized, and unable to group into a political force. Suffering is anchored in the human body, and to live amidst sufferers does not make it less miserable for the individual, but underprivileged communities are more visible targets for redistribution than individuals.

Recognition can be seen as the opposite of neglect, that is, neglect must be made visible before moving on to recognition of the individual's identity, moral standing and social participation. Although both recognition and redistribution are intimately intertwined and oriented towards social justice, there can be no redistribution unless the sufferers of injustice or discrimination are identified and sufficiently empowered to state their case. Redistribution can only follow after the harms of misrecognition have been corrected The ethics of recognition blends naturally with contemporaneous cultural concerns with personal identity, capabilities and empowerment: "Because it destroys an essential presupposition of the individual's capability to act, every moral injury represents an act of personal harm" (Honneth 1995, 9).

## IX. IDENTITY

Contemporary scholars divide their attention between the psychological importance of recognition to build and maintain "harmonious or flourishing personal identities and self-conceptions", the social dimension solidifying and ethically improving the interaction of people as peers but also respecting the differences and, thirdly, the political struggle for multicultural recognition and equality (Laitinen and Ikäheimo 2011). These three aspects are firmly intertwined for the purpose of addressing the issues of neglect.

Personal identity is a prime example of estrangement between philosophy and individuals living in the world where selfhood is an elementary feature of every human being. The self-conscious reality of personal identity, in terms of belonging to a group that issues a membership acknowledgement and as the singular person one is, has come under attack.

> Whether in their consciousness or their subconscious, men and women of our times are haunted by the *specter of exclusion*. They are

*Rights and Justice* 31

aware –as Hauke Brunkhorst poignantly reminds us– that millions have already been excluded, and that for 'those who fall outside the functional system, be it in India, Brazil or Africa, or even as at present in many districts of New York or Paris, all others soon become inaccessible. Their voices will no longer be heard, often they are literally struck dumb'. (Bauman 2005, 47)

Identity must reinvent itself as individual existence changes. Identities are reinvented as people migrate, change neighborhood, take on new jobs or become unemployed. Chronic disease requires the adaptation of a previously healthy identity, modified familial status provokes an identity crisis as do severe losses. Identity requires marking in participation and differentiation with its new agenda of rights and duties.

Relationality with significant others begins with love and care for the dependent and powerless child, creating and cultivating more distant social interactions based on the adscription, membership, and participative interaction of the individual sculpting an identity that needs to be recognized in order to authenticate the claim of belonging to a community and exercising the moral and civil capabilities of citizenship.

We need relationships, and we need relationships in which we count for something, relationships to which we can refer in order to define ourselves. But because of the long-term commitments which they notoriously inspire or inadvertently spawn, relationships may be, in a liquid modern environment, fraught with dangers. (Bauman 2005, 68)

Contemporary psychologists will insist that recognition precedes cognition: babies first recognize that they are being cared for and loved before having cognitive awareness of their surroundings. Social and political recognition are more sophisticated processes obscuring the basic role of moral recognition that secures individual identity and inspires the struggle for such purported universals as human dignity, the intrinsic value of human life, and the equal moral value of human groups too often discriminated against. The politics of recognition includes the feature of universalism, but also that of recognizing difference and uniqueness:

Our identity is partly shaped by the recognition or its absence, often by the *mis*recognition of others, and so a person or group of people can suffer real damage, real distortion, if the people or society around them mirror back a confining or demeaning or contemptible picture of themselves. Nonrecognition or misrecognition can inflict harm, can be a form of oppression, imprisoning, someone in a false, distorted, and reduced mode of being. (Taylor 1995, 225)

Even more important is the complex process of moral recognition, which is the tragedy of those who have no opportunity to obtain the moral recognition required to integrate as a member of society. The pervasive lack of recognition is overshadowed by more harmful acts of active misrecognition suffered by so many human beings, that prevails not only among the poor and marginal, but also in the midst of societies revolving in an unceasing roundabout of production and consumption, where persons are merely identified as working units without a face; unhinged from experiential private life they resurface as manipulated consumer units, causing pathologies of the self –overloaded narcissism, fatigue of self, and self-alienation– (Han 2015). "The meaning of the 'underclass identity' is an *absence of identity*; the effacement or denial of individuality, of 'face' – that object of ethical duty and moral care" (Bauman 2005, 39).

## X. EMPOWERMENT AND CAPABILITIES

Confirming identity and having it morally recognized are a first step towards actually existing in the world with others, requiring a certain set of capabilities and empowerment to struggle for continued recognition, claim one's rights and perform as a citizen.

The "Capability Approach" favored by Amartya Sen, and the "capability theory of justice" developed by Martha Nussbaum, are based on a concept of the set of valuable "beings and doings" that empowers people to seek in liberty their values and options to realize their preferred way of life. Capabilities are necessary to freely opt for a "good life" –Sen–

*Rights and Justice* 33

which, in Nussbaum's lexicon means pivoting around a theory of justice respectful of human dignity. Sen aims at enhancing individual freedom, and Nussbaum's theory is founded on respecting human dignity –self-respect, "nonhumiliation" and equality–, developed to achieve a flourishing life. Though touching on recognition, the Capability Approach speaks of development and achievement whereas the ethics of recognition first of all applies to the avoidance and correction of misrecognitions and the dire consequences of suffering and neglect. Freedom and self-respect ought to allow the unhindered display of capabilities, that is, "vectors of functioning, reflecting the person's freedom to lead one type of life or another" (Sen 1995, 40). Capabilities are engines that need to be stimulated, they are functional capacities that require empowerment to achieve results, and the poor may be disempowered to a degree that hinders the exercise of basic capabilities. Income poverty lines fail to relate levels of income with the empowerment to exercise basic capabilities: "So the focus of attention of poverty analysis has to be capability as opposed to achievement" (Ibid., 112).

Social empowerment is a broad area of practice drawing upon social work and communal development principles. Social empowerment is typically implemented at four stages: (1) the individual level –where the person values him/herself and actively wants to participate in life, (2) the family level, (3) the community level, and (4) the social policies level impacting local and national level actions to promote social equity and the inclusion of all persons.

The insufficiency of capabilities devoid of the necessary empowerment to achieve is clearly illustrated by looking at the obstacles of availability and access that plague healthcare disparities and neglect. A medical service may be available but not accessible due to financial, geographic or other factors that conspire to hinder reaching for what is needed. Scarcity and a flourishing black market are vivid examples of how reduced availability creates massive inaccessibility.

The capabilities approach is well suited to a consensual approach, but
a politics of need should be about struggle, not consensus: the struggle for

the recognition of unspoken needs; the struggle for more direct forms of political participation; the struggle against exploitation and the systemic injustices of capitalism. (Dean 2009, 261)

*Chapter 2*

# MEDICINE IN HEALTH AND DISEASE

## I. ON HEALTH AND DISEASE

The production and accumulation of data nowadays exceed by far our actual knowledge and understanding of the human body's biological processes. Similarly, clinical exploration is much more elaborate and sophisticated than its therapeutic relevance, as can be easily confirmed by a brief look at infectious diseases: research in microbiology, virology and infectiology has been very productive, whereas the track record of antibiotics and antiviral agents is comparatively poor: effective, nontoxic and affordable new antibiotics have been few and short-lived, owing to the unsettling development of resistant microorganisms. Hence the undaunted fear of emergent and re-emergent infectious diseases, and the alarm at possible bouts of pandemics.

The swiftly changing spectrum of diseases, therapies, public health policies and biomedical practices, upsets what two generations ago was the historical tradition of medicine and the bequest it used to pass on to fledgling healthcare practitioners: the heritage of knowledge, of tradition, ethics and behavior and, thirdly, of problems: "We must distinguish, however, between the continuity of the problems and the variations in the answers. The answers change; the problems, the questions, remain the same" (King 1982, 9–10).

Rapid and profound changes put these views in question, especially the idea that the problems of medicine remain unchanged. Without going further, middle- and high-income societies have taken part in the epidemiological turn from infectious diseases towards a predominance of non-communicable diseases, while poor populations continue to suffer and die from parasitic, bacterial and viral diseases. The problem of infections is a host/pathogen imbalance inflamed by unfavorable environmental factors; degenerative non-communicable chronic conditions respond to multiple causes including the almost ineffable "unhealthy lifestyle" (Sastya et al. 2018).

The problems of medical and healthcare are compounded since the concepts of health, disease, and disability are becoming increasingly discretional, changing their existential and social meaning, and creating a two-world medical reality: hyperactive medicalization and disease mongering among the better-situated, and neglect and indolence for the poor.

## II. HEALTH

The common belief and practice that health is the absence of disease have been overturned by the World Health Organization's proclamation that "health is a state of complete physical, mental and social well-being and not merely the absence of disease or infirmity." If so, the condition of health is nonexistent.

In 1986 the WHO presented the Ottawa Charter for Health Promotion, which does not modify the holistic and unrealistic original definition of health:

> Health promotion is the process of enabling people to increase control over, and to improve, their health. To reach a state of complete physical mental and social wellbeing, an individual or group must be able

# Medicine in Health and Disease

to identify and to realize aspirations, to satisfy needs, and to change or cope with the environment. Health is, therefore, seen as a resource for everyday life, not the objective of living. Health is a positive concept emphasizing social and personal resources, as well as physical capacities. Therefore, health promotion is not just the responsibility of the health sector, but goes beyond healthy lifestyles to wellbeing.

The Conference calls on the World Health Organization and other international organizations to advocate the promotion of health in all appropriate forums and to support countries in setting up strategies and programmes for health promotion.

The Conference is firmly convinced that if people in all walks of life, nongovernmental and voluntary organizations, governments, the World Health Organization and all other bodies concerned join forces in introducing strategies for health promotion, in line with the moral and social values that form the basis of this CHARTER, health for all by the year 2000 will become a reality.

The self-assured optimism of such documents surely did not consider that neglected populations also ought to reach "health for all" within 15 years. These WHO proclamations have been amply criticized for being of little practical value, and not accountable. They remain canonical for teaching purposes, and for a few scholars who enjoy the verbosity of holistic rhetoric. Some criticisms are negative for the wrong reasons: "It [the WHO definition] minimises the role of the human capacity to cope autonomously with life's ever changing physical, emotional, and social challenges and to function with fulfilment and a feeling of wellbeing with a chronic disease or disability" (Huber et al. 2011, 2). In this view, human beings have the empowerment to cope, reach fulfillment and attain wellbeing. Far from having universal reach, this definition deepens the cleft between the "empowered to cope" and those who, lacking the capabilities to do so, remain invisible and neglected.

The French neurosurgeon René Leriche (1879-1995) briefly stated that "Health is life lived in the silence of the organs", a dictum taken up in the lucid and well-known writings of George Canguilhem (1904-1955), and recently commented on by *The Lancet*'s editor-in-chief, who adds: "Health cannot be seen or touched or known. Health lies outside our perception" (Horton 2012, 961). Ubiquitously employed, health is an ineffable concept, a non-experience, and therefore of little practical use to plan medical and public "health" programs of any kind, while the much touted right to health remains devoid of any meaning whatsoever.

In daily life people are healthy in terms of being unaware that their body is unobtrusively functioning in for them a normal way. Medicine and public health have taken care to warn us that this is a state of pseudo-health that needs to be perforated by finely-tuned diagnostic instruments that will, more often than not, reveal genetic anomalies, predispositions, and risk factors, prescribing preventive individual improvements of lifestyle and permanent medical surveillance. Slogans like healthcare, the right to health, healthy living, and learning to cope and be resilient, fall on the complacent ears of those who are not plagued by basic needs, nourishing medicalization, "healthism" and lucrative enterprises promoting healthy lifestyles.

The science of genetics has effectively blurred the limits between health and disease. The initial idea of discovering a one-to-one match between genetic alterations and specific diseases –one gene one disease, one gene one enzyme– has been shown to be an oversimplification of complex molecular processes where genes within a genome have multiple interactions, and are subject to external influences after birth. These complex and as yet little-known processes will co-determine whether, when and how genetic abnormalities may express themselves as diseases.

The so-called "new public health" or risk epidemiology has insistently positioned the prevention of disease and the promotion of health as each person's responsibility, urged to attend regular medical check-ups, and adjust their lifestyle to engage in healthy nutrition, physical exercise and the avoidance of unhealthy sedentary habits. People are nudged to consume health and be aware of quaternary preventivism –the avoidance of iatrogenic preventive medicine, excessive medicalization, and coping with the oxymoron of being a healthy patient.

Efforts at promoting health and preventing disease notwithstanding, common sense and everyday medical practice continue to maintain a

# Medicine in Health and Disease

pragmatic description of health as the absence of disease: health checks, child health, and healthy ageing. The overlapping concepts of healthcare and medical care lead to confusion when, for example, a right to health or a right to medical care at a "primary", "decent minimum" level is not clearly disambiguated. Populations that live in dire conditions are prone to neglected diseases that lack access to medical treatment, and healthcare disparities manifest themselves as unequal medical attention ranging from excessive medicalization for the privileged, to a total absence of medical services, a range within which it becomes impossible to situate a decent minimum of medical care.

It might be useful to combine the notion of health with Martha Nussbaum's previously mentioned work on identifying a range of "central human functional capabilities", a list of 10 items, the first three of which are: the capability for physical survival, the capability for bodily health, the capability for bodily integrity (Nussbaum 1999). In later elaborations, these basic corporeal capabilities become culturally diluted: life worth living, bodily health –being able to have good health–, and bodily integrity –move freely, be secure, have opportunities for sexual satisfaction and for choice in matters of reproduction– (Nussbaum 2011). In the first version, health is lost when corporeal capabilities are hampered by bodily dysfunction; the second version concedes that a life worth living is the privilege of minorities.

## III. ILLNESS, DISEASE AND THE CLINICAL ENCOUNTER

Though often employed as interchangeable descriptions of maladies affecting the human organism, feeling ill and having a disease are distinct concepts. Illness is the feeling of being unwell beyond the controllable and self-limited misery of conditions like morning sickness, motion sickness, a bout of flu or other forms of temporarily feeling under the weather. Phenomenologists like to say that feeling ill pertains to the lived body experiencing how the living body is in an uncontrollable state of disorder, which prompts seeking therapeutic alleviation. The ill person consults a physician –or other trustworthy therapeutic agent– when suffering an unrelenting bodily disorder of upsetting, even alarming intensity and duration.

Traditionally, illness becomes disease when symptoms and signs can be classified within a medically and socially accepted nosology –taxonomy of disorders–. "Diagnostic exploration of a patient's condition has as its primary goal to intervene and [positively] change this condition... Securing a diagnosis without any consequence is unprofessional medical practice" (Wieland 1975, 69, 90). This sound explanation seems forgotten in current biomedical efforts, where genetic findings pose early preclinical conditions, and disease categories are inspired and medicalized according to vested interests, the human body explored without an intention to clarify possible therapeutic measures.

Certainly, the diagnostic workup has a number of other worthy functions like increasing medical knowledge, improving clinical experience, fortifying nosology and significant statistics, but all these goals should not ignore the primary medical objective of palliating and curing the patient's suffering. A critical view of current biomedical practices in Western culture needs to be resurfaced in view of the distortion of health/disease issues, and the influence of healthism, medicalization and pharmaceuticalization in the wake of growing healthcare disparities and a lack of medical services in neglected populations.

Pre-technical clinical diagnosis, though preliminary, serves the function of recognizing the disease by acknowledging the ill-feeling person's identity. This interplay between narrative and trust is perceptively described by John Berger in *A Fortunate Man* at a time when our culture witnesses the virtual collapse of the clinical encounter. As medical practice becomes impersonal –telemedicine–, the healthcare vision of the distant diseased turns blurred, indifferent and neglectful. "Self-perceived categories to represent disease, such as explanatory models or illness narratives, are extremely important, because they make present the connection between individual bodies and social bodies" (Das 1999, 126).

The clinical encounter is the traditional space where the ill-feeling individual seeks the advice and therapeutic intervention of the physician; it

*Medicine in Health and Disease* 41

is the classical venue of interpersonal medical practice. Much of today's dissatisfaction with contemporary medicine stems from the various forms in which this space shrinks and shrivels: brief consultation time, dismissal of patients' narrative, physical examination replaced by technical explorations, regulations set up by managed care or by underfinanced public health services, marketing strategies, and professional ethics transgressions posed as transparent and innocuous conflicts of interests. Scientific biomedicine delivers facts that square as poorly with patients' individual idiosyncrasy and values as they do with the doctor's experience and clinical acumen.

The problematic interface between Western biomedicine and policies aimed at the poor that are part of neglected populations, has been insufficiently highlighted by anthropological studies, that are beginning to explore how different cosmologies may well be a major factor explaining why technical solutions for neglected diseases are less efficacious than expected: "we find a mélange of categories, drugs, and practices, which make it impossible to distinguish between the 'native' categories of health and illness and the 'imposed' categories of biomedicine" (Ibid., 122).

# IV. MEDICALIZATION

Medicalization has been defined as a process by which non-medical problems are construed as medical issues falling under the jurisdiction of medicine. Michel Foucault traces medicalization back to the 18th century, as state, urban and industrial medicine successively developed a wide and dense network of medical practices. His ideas on the subject were presented in conferences delivered in Brazil (1974), at a time when Europeans were enjoying strong and lavish welfare states –Britain's National Health Service was a robust 30-year-old state institution providing healthcare "from cradle to grave"–, and Third World states were compelled to seek financial loans from the Bretton Woods institutions –the World Bank and the International Monetary Fund–. Under the "Washington consensus" countries receiving these loans were required to

# 42                                    *Miguel Kottow*

plan fiscal austerity and the privatization of public services, including medical care. As medicine became a marketable commodity –especially in issues of mental health and behavior "disorders"–, medicalization vastly expanded under the leadership of biomedical research, disease mongering, and the possessiveness of industrial giants commanding the pharmaceutical and medical devices markets.

Medicalization is directed at individual problems rather than at the "social environment", shunning "more collective or social solutions". Engineered by the pharmaceutical industry, human differences are transformed into diseases (Conrad 2007). The technoscientific impact on medicine has led to the more sophisticated process of biomedicalization.

> Biomedicalization describes the increasingly complex, multisited, multidirectional processes of medicalization, both extended and reconstituted through the new social forms of highly technoscientific biomedicine.
>
> Five key interactive processes both engender biomedicalization and are produced through it: (1) the political economic reconstruction of the vast sector of biomedicine; (2) the focus on health itself and the elaboration of risk and surveillance biomedicines; (3) the increasingly technological and scientific nature of biomedicine; (4) transformations in how biomedical knowledges are produced, distributed, and consumed, and in medical information management; and (5) transformations of bodies to include new properties and the production of new individual and collective technoscientific identities. (Clarke et al. 2003, 161)

Nowhere is the deep cleft between social groups and individuals so wide and visible as in the clinical encounter expanded and dominated by the self-management of health promotion and disease prevention –new public health, the Ottawa Charter–, sustained by "health literacy" and achieved thorough "health education" (WHO 1986; Nutbeam 2000).

A host of sociological studies have confirmed how core concepts like health, disease, medical therapy, as well as public health and healthcare jargon are modified and construed by corporate interests led by the pharmaceutical giants, endlessly extending medical jurisdiction without major concerns for all those who get marginalized, unattended and neglected by these pervasive practices. At the core of these practices –that make people sick, and are morally sickening– is rampant disease mongering.

As medicalization expands in consumer societies, the practice of medicine tends to replace the traditional patient/physician relationship by relying on instrumental parameters to redefine health and disease, at the cost of sacrificing the more personal approach of narrative medicine, the widespread dismissal of the patient's experience of illness and the relevance of the medical humanities. Impoverished interpersonal relationships replaced by high-tech performances cannot be adapted to settings of absolute or even relative poverty.

# V. Disease Mongering

Mongering has lost its old-fashioned meaning of peddling, now resurfacing as a negative or harmful way of displaying or promoting something –warmongering–. Disease mongering is a newcomer to the market, referring to a number of activities aimed at "the selling of sickness that widens the boundaries of illness in order to grow markets for those who sell and deliver treatment" (Monynihan, Doran and Henry 2008). Disease mongering strategies vary from creating new disease entities, promoting the off-label use of registered drugs, aggravating mild problems into diseases, lowering the thresholds for treatment, expanding and exaggerating risk factors, creating incentives for multi-drug prescriptions, and indulging in sloppy or biased research.

The major agent in disease mongering is the pharmaceutical industry spending substantially more money on promotion than on R&D, as it distributes incentives to prescribing physicians, supports medical teaching and research institutes, and exerts strong lobbying to find favor with regulative and legislative instances, as well as influencing public health policies. The WHO's sweeping definition of mental health includes "subjective well-being, perceived self-efficacy, autonomy, competence, inter-generational dependence, and self-actualization of one's intellectual and emotional potential, among others." Alarmed by its estimates, that close to half of the world's population is affected by some sort of mental health problem, the WHO established its Mental Health Observatory, contributing to the lucrative marketing of mood stabilizers and boosters that continues to boom.

Cause-effect relations in health issues involved in the to-and-fro juggling of opinions, data, and colliding interests are as good as impossible to evaluate. Public health policies will support efforts at the prevention of maladies and the promotion of health, without sufficient cost/benefit evidence, often remaining oblivious to the fact that their feasibility, relevance and impact differ in diverse socioeconomic contexts. There are those who support any effort to increase public awareness of prevention and early diagnosis –"I am a disease monger. I teach primary care doctors how to identify bipolar disorder" (James Phelps)–, others state that "by protecting industry, not the public –the FDA is a purveyor of the psychiatric 'disease' and 'chemical imbalance' lie" (Fred Baughman); still others point out that "Promoting a particular body image or behaviour pattern as the preferred one and then selling medicines or products to help people attain the particular ideal may be regarded as disease mongering" (Shankar, Giri and Palaian). All these citations are taken from brief notes published in the *PloSMedicine* series on disease mongering in 2006, the final article putting matters in context with the realities of medical care disparities:

> There is some evidence of complacency about disease mongering on the part of regulators. The US Food and Drug Administration's recent proposal to relax restrictions on off-label marketing risked setting the conditions for disease mongering to flourish…Unnecessary medicalization and medication may be wasting precious health resources, with obvious opportunity costs for private and public insurers alike. (Moynihan, Doran and Henry 2006)

In a world where medicalization, disease mongering and neglected diseases coexist, the ideas of global ethics, universal human rights and generally shared values find no common ground for deliberation.

*Chapter 3*

# STRATEGIES OF BIOMEDICAL RESEARCH

## I. RESEARCH AND THE RELIABILITY OF INFORMATION

The modern world is pervaded by trust in science as the systematic study of reality by observation and experimentation. Scientific endeavors are based on facts yielding data that gain the status of reliable knowledge if consistently reproduced, statistically evaluated and coherently theorized.

Knowledge gained by methodic scientific research, we are told, is invariably correctable and deemed useful inasmuch as it is not polluted by opinions derived from non-scientific sources like ethics, theology, or philosophy, unless they too deign to become empirical explorers. Scientific results are translated into technical innovations that deliver novel instruments to science, explaining the current use of the term technoscience, expanding into a self-induced and self-regulated gigantic enterprise, feeding a consumer society that drives the supply and demand market to extremes of sophistication, and increasing discrimination and inequality between the solvent and the impecunious.

Trust in technoscience opens the way to technocracy, a political system where experts occupy powerful positions in social institutions and government. Technocrats are decision-makers based on facts and aimed at specific, empirically measurable goals –growth, unemployment, and inflation–, impervious to problems of conflicting values and interests (Evans 2006). Technocracy is the triumph of pragmatic reasoning, disenchanting the world by applying science and enlightened reason to investigate and control every nook and cranny of reality.

The first clouds are obscuring technoscientific complacency as the high ecological price to be paid by progress comes into view, and awareness grows that well-being reaches a minority of human beings. The optimism that technoscience will resolve its own deficiencies is no longer credible, given that it caters to a consumer society that dismisses the rampant social and ecological problems in need of urgent attention.

As scientific research increasingly emphasizes investigations in biology, medicine, biomedicine and biotechnology, it slowly dawns that some critical sociology and ethical supervision is necessary. Sociologists have also insisted that scientific production is oblivious to social value and relevance, ignoring grassroots participation in research policies and priorities. Views from ethics worry that economic priorities are stifling nonmaterial values of self-respect, social cohesion and what Weber called *Wertrationalität* –value/belief-oriented rationality–, and what Habermas presents as communicative reason.

## II. BIOMEDICAL RESEARCH

Biomedicine has bowed to positivism by centering on the body as a repairable machine with replaceable organs –organ transplants, prostheses–. There seems to be no limit to redesigning the human body, as illustrated by a currently developing project on head transplant –head-exchange between two bodies–, known formally as the "Human Head Anastomosis Venture" (HEAVEN), announced to be performed in a living human being by early 2019. At the microlevel, relentless deconstruction of the organismproceeds to explore its molecular components –genes, enzymes– and their interactions –neural networks–. Fragmented biology is amenable to multiple experimental entry-points that result in a gigantic expansion of research, energizing irrelevant and redundant data collections to the tune of corporative and academic interests that ignore needs and benefits for the common weal, and often misguiding healthcare issues.

In the wake of the increasing costs of healthcare and medical services, governments have resorted to cost containment by reducing public financing and demanding empirical evidence of pharmaceutical drugs and medical devices, as practiced by such institutions as Britain's National Institute for Clinical Excellence –NICE–, and generally adopted by managed healthcare providers. In medical practice, evidence-based medicine has also fueled research to demonstrate the effectiveness and favorable benefit/cost relation of many therapeutic actions, though surveys show that general practitioners prefer to rely on experience and clinical acumen.

Disease research requires a great amount of basic investigation carried out by universities and research institutes that concentrate professional skills, equipment, and library facilities. The competitive world of academia nurtures a "reward culture that focuses excessively on papers and patents, and not on whether the research actually benefits society" (Butler 2007, 158). Consequently, basic R&D for neglected and rare diseases has little purchase in the highly specialized field of molecular biological investigation. Very slowly, some initiatives are being created to enhance the social value of research, including the exceptional promotion of free licensing at the University of California, Berkeley –considered a "moral compass"–, and Welcome Trust funds to support university-based research on neglected tropical diseases (NTDs).

The ideal of developing R&D sites in low- and middle-income countries that have local and regional needs for new drugs, has been fulfilled in only a handful of nations yielding isolated but notable results, such as Cuba developing a vaccine against a strain of *Neisseria*-induced meningitis, and the production of a hepatitis B vaccine in South Africa. On the whole, though, R&D in less developed countries is dominated by a strong North-South asymmetry (Singer et al. 2007).

Academia has been co-opted by the knowledge industry directed by big publishing companies, which impose their interests by multiplying specialized journals mainly filled with work by the chosen few Anglophone scholars. Basic research is being involved in corporative interests dictating what is to be investigated and how to publish its supportive results.

The money carousel of academia includes authors' fees for publishing in open-access journals, and the temptations of mushrooming predatory journals and books. Whichever way one looks at it, academia has to a large extent become an interests pampering machine in highly selective mainstream publications. Even such reputed institutions as the Cochrane Library have been reportedly involved in direct and indirect conflicts of interest.

Very few academic research facilities can apply basic knowledge gained in the laboratory to the complex strategies required to engage in application studies, which in biomedicine are essentially clinical trials. If a basic investigation happens to be promising, further research aiming at a clinical application will be taken over by the pharmaceutical industry, especially if the final product is expected to be a patentable drug that will generate substantial profits, perhaps even hit the jackpot of a blockbuster with sales in the billions. A habitual procedure is for Big Pharma to buy promising basic research patents and engage in the successive phases of clinical research protocols, mounting or contracting a complex network of research centers to glide through the phases of clinical research: Phase I investigates safety and toxicity levels in healthy volunteers, Phase II engages patients to study effectiveness, and Phase III is a large-scale clinical study to determine safety, effectiveness and appropriate dosages.

The development of drugs and vaccines for neglected diseases yields products that need to be low-priced and accessible to impoverished populations, which are not adequately subsidized in low-income countries, as well as to middle-income patients with only patchy reimbursement schemes.

*Strategies of Biomedical Research*            51

## III. RESEARCH REGULATIONS AND GUIDES

Biomedical research entails the risks of harm and exploitation that ought to be minimized or avoided by complying with guidelines and declarations concerning the correctness of professional ethics, and subject protection overseen by bioethics.

The quest for a bridging tie between hard sciences and the humanities – C. P. Snow and Van Renselaer Potter– has not been honored. In fact, the academic presence of the humanities is declining, and the two cultures' distinction is triangulated by the emergence of the social sciences that have introduced the paradigm of qualitative research, though they are bent on being validated as quantitative empirical science, thus weakening their original connection with the humanities, including critical theory, human values studies, ethics and bioethics.

The development and institutionalization of ethical requirements in research involving human beings, as well as nonhuman animals, have been rapidly evolving as the aftermath of brutal experiments performed during the German fascist regime (1933-1945), beginning with the Nuremberg Code (1948), followed by the Helsinki Declaration (1964) and its successive revisions, the Guidelines of CIOMS, Good Medical Practices, and hosts of national and regional declarations. The American Belmont Report (1979) formally mandated that research protocols were to be approved by ethics committees –Institutional Research Boards–, with special emphasis on securing voluntary informed consent to participate as research subjects, and including a growing number of requirements concerning risks, undesirable side effects, and benefits, all in all leading to debates and regulations aiming at international scientific and ethical standards of clinical research.

The first Declaration of Helsinki (1964) explicitly stated:

> Medical progress is based on research which ultimately must rest in part on experimentation involving human subjects. In the field of biomedical research a fundamental distinction must be recognised between medical research in which the aim is essentially diagnostic or

therapeutic for a patient, and medical research the essential object of which is purely scientific and without implying direct diagnostic or therapeutic value to the person subjected to the research.

The "fundamental distinction" between therapeutic and non-therapeutic –"purely scientific"– was dismissed by researchers claiming that every treatment has an experimental side to it, while every clinical trial has therapeutic value. The distinction was dropped in later versions of the Helsinki Declaration, boosting the offshoring practice of recruiting subjects for trials that had no medical value for them. It was repeatedly claimed that patients who lacked mental competence to give informed consent should nevertheless not be excluded from clinical trials, improperly incorporating them in non-therapeutic studies including possible unwanted side effects to which they were subject. Normative weaknesses are detected, for example, when non-therapeutic research is done in incompetent individuals, arguing that the "minimal" risks involved are acceptable even if voluntary consent is unavailable.

In this initial version of 1964, the Declaration of Helsinki also stated, that "At the conclusion of the study, every patient entered into the study should be assured of access to the best proven prophylactic, diagnostic and therapeutic methods identified by the study." This paragraph (originally No. 30) has been actively contended, revised and watered down in more recent versions, resulting in the practice that post-trial benefits are denied more often than not by arguing that the investigated drug needs further studies and has yet to be approved and registered. In any event, the argument goes on, post-trial benefits that might extend for many years, are beyond the costs that research sponsors purportedly could afford. Contended issues like the use of placebos in control groups, or doing research in communities that will not have the benefit of any "local social value", all point towards the powerful pressure of corporate interests disregarding ethical requirements that they see as hampering their expansive self-interested policies.

International guidelines for ethics in research with human beings have progressively reduced their initial motivation of protecting research

# Strategies of Biomedical Research 53

subjects from unethical and abusive procedures, and requiring unrestricted respect for their autonomy by honoring voluntary and well-informed consent to participate. These instruments seek international approval by employing a noncommittal verbose style, and suggesting a discretional consideration of their norms.

More than half a century of declarations, international documents and conventions, has yielded an immense corpus of pro/con publications, ranging from enthusiastic support (Andorno 2007), to explicit doubts about their legitimacy (Schucklenk 2015). Due to the variety of stakeholders that participate in the elaboration and implementation of research regulations, these proclamations necessarily employ a language bland enough to obtain a noncommittal consensus. Agents representing research interests outnumber those ensuring the protection of persons being included as research subjects, usually underprivileged –vulnerable– communities, and sick and dependent patients –clinical trials– often inexperienced in receiving medical care –therapeutically naive–. The pro research bias, including the vested interests of corporative sponsors, mostly the pharmaceutical industry acting directly or by hiring CROs, exerts influence to weaken protective clauses aimed at reducing harm and securing benefits for trial subjects. Normative issues are increasingly subject to discretional interpretation that resorts to loopholes such as non-therapeutic research in infants when "minimal risks" are involved, employing placebos when supported by "compelling scientific reasons", or promising post-trial benefits "if reasonably possible".

The consensus-seeking spirit of these normative efforts brings to light watered-down discourses carefully worded to avoid stepping on the toes of the mighty, where dealing with the contentious issues of neglected and rare diseases is most unlikely to reach the agenda. R&D is responsive to market value rather than actual health needs and a hallmark of the lack of strong social commitment of pharma giants, disguised by goodwill declarations, acts of donation, occasional patent sharing and voluntarily renouncing market exclusivity, all sparsely doled out and tailored so as to avoid cutting into profits. The research, production and sale of medicines continue to be splendidly profitable enterprises, allowing the industry to save face by donations and the selective sacrifice of patent advantages, always remaining insistently loyal to their shareholders who expect to remain profitable at all costs.

A recent press release (Health and Lifestyle Dec. 11, 2017) reports about a 9-year-old boy suffering from a painful skin disease –junctional epidermolysis bullosa– resistant to all known treatments, who is cured by a never-before-employed experimental gene therapy. This case illustrates how hopeless clinical situations merit, but almost never attain, access to promising drugs still in the research phase. Patients suffering from advanced disease, where no therapy exists, who are at risk of severe irreversible deterioration and death, are candidates to become research subjects in protocols that are in Phase I of clinical trial –experimental therapy–, off-trial experimental therapy, accelerated and expedited approval regulation, compassionate medicine. Because these approaches are essentially subject to the ethics of biomedical research with human beings, a fine-grained analysis is essential: placebos have no place in crucial experimental therapy nor should beneficial results of these preliminary trials be withheld from severely affected patients who, having participated in the study, ought to continue receiving therapeutic relief for as long as medically indicated. Access to experimental therapies is far from straightforward due to the strictness of inclusion criteria, rejected patients resorting to the request of compassionate medicine that, in turn, is subject to rigorous regulation and, in the end effect, to the willingness of the producers to provide the unavailable but promising drug. Thus, important drugs may exist but be unavailable due to impassable access restrictions imposed by manufacturers.

# IV. THE PHARMACEUTICAL INDUSTRY

The pharma industry has been increasing its profits by an annual average of 15% while the profit market of non-drug companies fluctuates in the 4-9% range. And yet, drug manufacturers are deeply concerned because revenues are falling as patents expire, new developments are slow

## Strategies of Biomedical Research 55

in coming, and research is more expensive. Regulatory requirements, it claims, are increasingly demanding and restrictive, while sales are slowed by costs containment in healthcare systems, and reduced out of pocket paying capacity. Nevertheless, the pharma giants continue to be among the most lucrative businesses in the world economy.

The pharma industry also claims that drug prices are high because R&D is costly. Research and Development (R&D) budgets, especially the latter, have gone up by 7%. Although money spent on research is tax deductible, research budgets amount to no more than one-third of expenditures on promotion. More importantly, R&D has yielded very few new drugs; most of those developed are so-called "me too" drugs, which are minor variations or new indications for products on the market, thus renewing for many years patent rights that are expiring (Angell 2005). Searching for new low-risk drugs that will be highly efficacious for at present untreatable diseases like multiple sclerosis, drug-resistant infections or emerging pathogens –Zika, Ebola– is time- and resource-consuming and, so the pharma industry predicts, will have a limited market for a number of reasons: the drugs developed will be expensive with a reduced sales potential; researching and producing vaccines for massive use will have to be unprofitably inexpensive, as they are incorporated into compulsory, yet precariously funded, vaccination programs aimed at obtaining herd immunity in areas with endemic infestation and threats of epidemic outbursts. When distant infections threaten to extend and affect the richer countries, as occurred with the HIV pandemic, research becomes active, generously funded, and anticipative of huge profits.

Protected by patents and monopoly-friendly policies, unwilling to innovate in prevention and therapy for diseases that affect the impecunious poor, the industry also fails to research treatment for rare diseases that, by definition, will only create a small market of unaffordable high-priced products –orphan drugs–. The pharma industry is the one major cause of inequalities in health; its profit avidity remains untouched by all relief and assistance programs devised to solve the availability of essential drugs. Notably the Health Impact Fund proposal (see, Chapter 7 IV-B) is careful to "give pharmaceutical innovators stable financial incentives to develop new medicines that have large effects on global health" (Banerjee, Hollis and Pogge 2010, 166).

## V. BIOMEDICAL RESEARCH IN RARE DISEASES

The research, production and marketing of diagnostic and therapeutic drugs for rare diseases show certain peculiarities that explain, and try to justify, the high market prices of these drugs, usually reaching several hundred thousand dollars yearly per patient, often without significant evidence of sustained benefits. Most therapeutic approaches are unique for each rare disease because the underlying genetic defect is not shared by other conditions, thus making precise diagnostic and narrowly focused treatment, a process fraught with difficulties, expenses and time-consuming research. These are the main reasons given by pharmaceutical companies to avoid venturing into this field and, if they do, to explain the enormous prices charged. Being a for-profit enterprise accountable to their shareholders, the pharma industry is impervious to ethical or social arguments suggesting policies that might sacrifice revenues.

The research and development of diagnostic and therapeutic agents for rare diseases are plagued by additional tensions, related to data accumulation, research strategies, benefits, and compassionate medicine. The extremely low prevalence of specific rare diseases may require culling data from many countries, a feat that Contract Research Organizations (CROs) claim to excel in. The repository of scarce data suggests that biobanks are the obvious tool for significant research into diseases with low prevalence.

Biobanks are defined by the Organization for Economic Co-operation and Development (OECD) as "a collection of biological material and the associated data and information stored in an organized system, for a population or a large subset of a population" (Graham et al. 2014, 50). Ethical and scientific standards are still in flux, and legislation is hesitant

# Strategies of Biomedical Research 57

and fragmentary facing some of the most debated features of biobanks: confidentiality, consent, international exchange and commercialization. Privacy and the need for biobank data for rare diseases are at unresolved odds (Mascalzoni, Paradiso and Hansson 2014).

There is a widespread feeling that orphan drugs should be available for all patients afflicted with a rare disease provided they are of some therapeutic value at least in slowing progression and postponing premature death, and that they be financed without cuts in other items of the healthcare budget (Aronson 2006). As an alternative to no treatment, orphan drugs are not to be withheld, but when more alternative therapies are available, a "comparative-effectiveness" form of metrics ought to be applied.

> More generally, scholars of health economics have advocated for the importance of comparative-effectiveness research in more efficiently allocating health resources –in particular in situations where it may be infeasible to use cost-efficacy as a decision metric. To this end, we recommend a metric that is developed transparently and through continued roundtable cooperation of patients, other tax payers, industry, insurance and EU governments with the above factors in mind, bearing in mind legal arguments which demand providing these measures. (Hyry, Stern, Roos and Cox 2014, 244)

Nothing in this quote suggests that the extremely high prices of drugs should be in any way discouraged or regulated. In fact, the authors state, somewhat ambiguously that "they are also 'expensive' because of the laudable legislative incentive schemes [market exclusivity] to remedy this problem" (Ibid., 242), a fairly unusual way of justifying exorbitant prices for necessary therapies. In a subsequent paper titled "Orphan Drugs: Expensive Yet Necessary" (Hyry, Roos and Cox, 2015), the authors seem to more readily accept the high price of drugs than if they had written "necessary yet expensive", a perhaps hair-splitting distinction, yet suggestive in view of the fairly long list of conflicts of interest involved.

# VI. COMMERCIALIZATION OF RESEARCH

Following Richard Merton's ideal of proper scientific commitment, "Mertorian Tories" consider science to be corrupted by commercialization, as opposed to "Economic Whigs" who believe economics' unavoidable influence on scientific work need not mar its correctness and reliability (Mirowski and Van Horn 2005). Increasingly, professional for-profit organizations have emerged that specialize in carrying out clinical studies; Contract Research Organizations (CROs) and Site Management Organizations (SMOs) have become instrumental in reinforcing patent policies developed and refined as the main strategy securing corporative profits at the cost of ignoring disease burdens among the less fortunate. CROs are now a major player in the commercialization of biomedical research and knowledge dissemination, having grown in a few decades from an obscure cottage industry into a multimillion enterprise that captures substantially more research business than the traditional university-based Academic Health Centers (AHCs). CROs promote their services to efficiently conduct clinical trials from inception to regulative registration, convincingly promising that their research costs are lower than those of the pharmaceutical industry, and that their strategies fill in stages where they have more expertise and international connections than their clients. One of the major CROs touts its knowhow in a promotional document titled "Overcoming Four Challenges to Successful Rare Disease Drug Development": "A firm understanding of how to navigate global regulatory environments is crucial to ensuring successful submission...accelerating market access for products that are aligned to payer and provider demands" (ICON, Pharmafocus, April 2017).

Ethical oversight of biomedical research in animals and human beings is mandatory, for many years exercised by Institutional Review Boards (IRBs) that, though overloaded to the point of hastiness, continue to pass binding judgments on the ethical aspects of the AHC's research. CROs have successfully lobbied to be reviewed by independent boards, hiring bioethics consultants, and generally reducing to a minimum disclosure of their activities. Conflicts of interests ensue, making it difficult to hold

*Strategies of Biomedical Research* 59

CROs "up to consistency and quality standards, together with the risks of noncompliance" (Mirowksi and Van Horn 2005, 513).

Even though CROs are barred from securing intellectual property by seeking patents, they provide tool kits that allow the biomedical industry to make lavish use of patent facilities not only for products, but also for processes of research. CROs excel at delivering marketable products, to which effect they expedite research and registration processes, actively participating in the preparation of publishable material that is needed to secure intellectual property. CROs support scientific publications by providing ghost writers, guest authors and "medical communications companies" that contribute to foster "academic publications [that] may be viewed, more often than not, as 'infomercials' that aid the marketing of the drug" (Ibid., 530).

Outsourcing biomedical research may be cost saving for the pharmaceutical industry, but the fact that CROs are thriving and expanding as big earner enterprises is instrumental in driving up the prices of end products that reach the market driven by adamantine intellectual protection practices. Commercialization of scientific projects is a continuous and growing tendency, that is successful enough to co-opt AHCs and university-based research activities. Needless to say, the immediate victims are rare diseases and neglected healthcare issues, which remain unattractive unless some breakthrough discovery brings to the market a product sellable at what critics call "outrageous prices" (Luzzatto et al. 2018). Abundant examples can be found of effective therapeutic drugs sold at patent-protected high prices that will produce revenues eight times higher than the R&D costs invested.

A medicine is not a consumer good that we can take or leave depending on price. The health profession has adhered to the moral imperative that, as long as there is an effective treatment for a patient with a certain disease, we must administer that treatment. For millennia human societies have translated moral imperatives into laws. (Luzzatto et al. 2015, 751)

# 60     Miguel Kottow

"Is there an effective policy to limit the prices faced by drug plans while still providing sufficient incentive to pharmaceutical companies to develop and market orphan drugs?" (Fellows and Hollis 2013, 180). The question leads to economic formulae searching for new approaches to cost containment, incentives, and regulated returns, all of which have been unable to mitigate, let alone solve the problem.

Risk-averting regulations require careful, thorough and significant evidence provided by clinical trials which ensure safety and efficacy that are at least equal, hopefully superior, to current medical treatments. Research procedures are lengthy, even considering the shortcuts taken by Big Pharma and CROs to avidly reach the market with prompt results. It has been suggested that provisional reimbursement should be based on preliminary favorable cost/effectiveness results and ongoing research, the result of which will confirm or withdraw financial support, in an effort to avoid reviewing new drugs while "condemning the victims of rare diseases to death" (Clarke 2006).

Pharmaceutical giants have developed four major strategies to protect their oligopolistic hegemony over the medical market, and pursue their narrow-minded R&D policies to increase profits unencumbered by social responsibility and reasonable accountability: patents and data exclusivity, the upkeep of the 10/90 gap, commercialization and outsourcing of R&D clinical trials buttressed by strategies to deviate the costs and burdens of research –offshoring research, hindering post-investigational benefits, and establishing double standards for research ethics–.

## VII. Patents and Data Exclusivity

Patents are safeguards of intellectual property, granting the patent-holder exclusive rights to the optional use of the registered property at his discretion, including the prevention of its use by others. The U.S. Patent and Trademark Office grants patents for useful, non-obvious and novel products and processes; the European Patent Office regulating many European countries, denies patents involving human embryonic stem cells.

Individual countries may deny patents to inventions that are contrary to their public's interest. France prohibits patents on "the human body, its elements, and its products, as well as knowledge of the total or partial structure of a human gene" (Johnston 2008, 94). Patent legislation varies from one country to another, there having been heavy discussions on the issue of patenting discoveries and inventions on the human body.

Patent registration is subject to strong lobbying influence and discretional, at times arbitrary, interpretations. The limited innovative capacity of the pharma industry has driven the registration of "me too" drugs that are little more than variations of products that are running out of patent, only needing to prove that they are effective: as effective or even less so than currently available drugs. The requirement of novelty is thus easily bypassed to renew a patent for another 20 years.

The World Trade Organization (WTO) was created in 1995, requiring all member states to sign the Agreement on Trade-related Aspects of Intellectual Property Rights (TRIPs) including the implementation of patent protection for pharmaceuticals. Powerful high-income countries' primary goal was to secure incentives –patents, market monopoly– for continued pharmaceutical innovation. "Developing" countries argued that the Agreement would hinder the local production of generic low-cost medicines, and provide additional support for the pharmaceutical industry to dominate the market with expensive products. Least Developed Countries (LDC) fought for a transitional period of 15 years to develop local R&D policies according to their own needs, an extension that was granted with the proviso that each country ought to negotiate its terms for the extension period on a case-by-case basis. A second Agreement was reached in 2001 known as the Doha Declaration, with the purpose of easing access restrictions, considering that it would take most LDCs a long time to reach the technical and economic independence to locally produce sufficient generic medicines to cover their populations' needs. The Brazilian experience has shown that productive local research for "technological, social and economic development" is only successful in countries with strong industrial infrastructure. Nations with underdeveloped production facilities cannot benefit from diligent local research, which finally goes to potent international enterprises (Morel et al. 2007).

The DOHA intends to support members' right to protect public health and promote access to medicines for all, aimed at clarifying the terms of a national health emergency that would lead to compulsory licenses and parallel imports (Correa 2002; Azam 2016).

Compulsory licensing is a TRIPs-recognized public health safeguard allowing a government to temporarily override a patent and authorize the production of generic versions of a patented product. Parallel importing occurs when the patent holder sells a product to a buyer who exports the product to a second buyer in another country. Such practice arises when, taking into account transportation and tariffs, the price of an elsewhere imported product, remains lower than the price of the same product legally made or imported into the country.

Compulsory licensing is also pursued in middle- and high-income countries bent on reducing high-priced drugs that neither the public health systems nor the average citizen could afford to pay. Legal battles are incensed by incoherent regulations in different countries, and by the interference of two separate regulatory systems: the intellectual property system basically concerned with patents, and the drug regulatory system that handles the registration system.

The aftermaths of DOHA and its multilateral approach to favor LDCs led high-income countries, under the influence of the U.S. and some European nations, to seek direct bilateral Free Trade Agreements (FTAs) imposing conditions and sanctions that canceled out DOHA's liberalities, by toughening requirements to apply for compulsory licenses and parallel imports. This post-DOHA situation, known as TRIPs plus, kept many countries from improving their healthcare situation, given that failing to comply by FTAs might lead to severe financial sanctions that the LDCs could not afford. A few nations, like Brazil and India, defied TRIPs plus restrictions based on their scientific and industrial power to manufacture generic equivalents.

# Strategies of Biomedical Research 63

While many believed the introduction of minimum standards and greater enforcement for intellectual property rights (IPRs) through the Agreement on Trade-Related Aspects of Intellectual Property (TRIPs) sufficiently placated the major industrialized nation's demand for strong IPRs, it now appears that this agreement only served as another step in the pursuit of stronger IPRs. (Mercurio 2006, 215)

The profusions of bilateral FTAs, which tend to benefit the stronger negotiating partner, end up by requiring new multilateral adjustments seeking more fairness between producers and consumers, investing time and efforts to accommodate the interests of the wealthy with the needs of the poor. At present, these efforts remain mostly *in spe*.

The...commitment of donors should be translated into resources to redress the inequities of financing, from which NTD programmes presently suffer, to give the poor what they deserve: access to free, high quality effective products as they continue to be exposed to an avoidable chronic pandemic which claimed at least ten-times more lives than the Ebola epidemic in a single year. (Moyneux, Savioli and Engels 2017, 32)

Patenting remains a crucial goal of R&D, aimed at securing profitable products from the interference of competitors. Given that patents are applied for some years before the product is registered and allowed to appear on the market, continuous efforts are displayed to extend the period of market exclusivity. Lower priced generics have only to prove their bioequivalence with the original product, shortcutting the registration procedure by using the clinical data provided by the original product, but the pharma industry has efficiently obstructed and delayed the development of generics, forcing more stringent FTAs that protect their interests by introducing data exclusivity obligations. Economic Western leaders have urged all countries to commit to a clear interpretation of TRIPs regulations that protect data from "unfair commercial use". The three reasons given for this drive to a more hermetic exclusivity are: a)

High revenues secure innovative research, and data exclusivity protects clinical data; b) Justice requires that data should not be available to "free-riders"; and c) Data exclusivity clauses should extend globally to include those nations that do not patent new biological drugs.

> Besides five years of data exclusivity for all new chemical entities, additional protection was granted for specific categories of drugs and clinical data. Where a new drug is recognized as an 'orphan drug' –for the treatment of rare conditions– a period of seven years of data exclusivity applies…As in the US, the EU has introduced a separate regime of ten years of data exclusivity for orphan drugs. (Diependaele, Cockbain and Sterckx 2017, 13)

A nonbiased critical analysis concludes that buttressing a market monopoly with data exclusivity is, to say the least, unfair. It "is inequitable and highly problematic to require developing countries to implement data exclusivity". From an ethical viewpoint, such regulations are simply perverse, "since current levels of revenue already generate copious profit margins for the pharmaceutical industry in US and EU markets" (Ibid., 21).

Data exclusivity has been harshened with the requirement that duly registered generic products cannot be marketed for ten years from the time the original product was put on the market, a ruling called market exclusivity. An additional delay may be imposed when the originator company files a new indication for its drug. Data and market exclusivity combine in a system known as the 8+2+1, allowing a maximum delay of 11 years before generics can enter the market. The market-dominated unavailability of orphan drugs could hardly be harsher.

# VIII. PATENTS AND PRICES

Big Pharma's generous distribution of medication and vaccines to care for NTDs, cannot hide its colossal monopoly as one of the largest profit-making enterprises in the current globalized economy (DeAngelis 2016).

*Strategies of Biomedical Research* 65

Year after year, statistics report high profit margins, which are disputed by the pharma industry as fake news. Scathing and well documented writings by Marcia Angell (2005) paint a murky picture of Big Pharma, including inflated bookkeeping on R&D tax-free expenditures, promotion budgets that exceed and at times more than double real R&D costs, the race for patenting non-innovative "me too" drugs, and other practices to ensure market-monopolies that drive drug prices above what insurances, public healthcare services, and private patients are willing or even able to pay: "Orphan drugs –those that treat small populations– are placing a substantial strain on the budgets of drug plans in many countries...Prices commonly exceed $100.000 per patient per year and are increasing" (Fellows and Hollis 2013; Luzzatto et al. 2015). Things become still more complicated when benefits/costs are evaluated with QALY criteria. The UK has ample experience through its National Institute for Health and Clinical Excellence (NICE), that approving a drug based on cost per QALY will create, as does any other form of rationing resources, a discriminating inclusion/exclusion divide.

The industry spends more than twice as much on promotion than on R&D. There is little transparency about the actual costs of researching and developing new drugs; suspicion has been raised that the black box of R&D hides expenses that go to marketing, and the costs of developing a new drug are claimed by the Pharmaceutical Research and Manufacturers of America to be substantially higher than most estimates. By inflating R&D costs, the drug industry justifies selling their products at high, in some instance exorbitant prices. Also, high costs save taxes.

Even after DOHA, "the current patent-based business model and the way we apply international patent rules need to change. The system is broke" (Ploumen and Schippers 2016, 339).

# IX. THE 10/90 GAP

In the early 1990s "the 10/90 gap" was "coined to convey the striking discrepancy identified between the size of disease burden and the allocation of health research funding" (Ramsay 2001, 1348; Luchetti 2014). As it stands, the gap often refers to the meager healthcare efforts that are devoted to the most disease-burdened populations, a claim that is at the base of all denunciations of healthcare inequities, forming the skeleton of global healthcare ethics and the quest for a more just social order. Healthcare disparities are condemnable because they fail to address treatable or preventable diseases, where effective medical agents exist but are not accessible to the poor, causing "unnecessary", avoidable deaths. Underlying this stark reality is that most R&D resources go to investigating the medical incommodities and problems that worry the small segment of high-income populations: 90% of all R&D efforts are funneled to medical conditions that affect the 10% more affluent section of the world population, by resorting to unnecessary me-too drugs, off-label indications that allow the renewal of patents, disease mongering and medicalization.

The specific problem of low priority R&D focused on diseases that have no effective preventive or therapeutic medical agents worsens healthcare inequity caused by maldistribution, poor access and availability affecting neglected populations.

The asymmetry between disease burdens and R&D priorities is inevitably furthered by market statistics: Over 80% of medical drugs consumption occurs in high-income countries (Europe, USA, Japan and the better-off minorities in Latin America). Africa and Asia, representing over 72% of world population, consume a meager 10% of available medicines. As China and India grow, these numbers may have to be revised, but the general trend remains unaltered.

Keeping the 10/90 gap open is supported by a number of research and market strategies that leave unattended endemic diseases affecting the poor, and those affected by rare diseases, combined with other tactics like offshoring and double-standard research ethics, access obstacles to experimental therapeutic research, and to compassionate medicine.

# X. Offshoring

Research initiatives are a key element of drug companies that are profitably positioned in the pharmaceutical market, permanently fuelled by the need to come up with new products as patents and monopoly strategies expire. The drive towards profitable novelty is a genuine search for more efficient substances expected to provide a therapeutic breakthrough and reach blockbuster sales. The quest for path-breaking originality is weary, extremely inefficient and costly, for medically useful innovations reach registration only rarely. A much-used alternative is to re-patent already registered drugs by making minor changes in their active principles, dosage or new indications, which makes them duplicates of existing products with the only purpose of getting into the market as "me too drugs" such as mood pills, non-steroidal anti-inflammatory drugs, psychopharmaca, multivitamins, and others.

In order to contain R&D costs in such a competitive market, drug producers and CROs have moved clinical trials to middle- and low-income countries –with a predilection for East European and Latin American research turfs– where labor and the installation of infrastructure are cheaper, and registration bureaucracy is easier to comply with. In addition, less developed countries have deficient healthcare facilities causing "treatment naivité" of populations that have had few previous interactions with therapeutic agents. It is tempting to apply pragmatic ethical standards in poor populations plagued by an abundance of "naïve subjects" –in its double meaning of subjects being less knowledgeable, but also unburdened by previous medications–. Research actively managed by CROs creates a double process of outsourcing: the pharma industry outsources to CROs, and these outsource by going offshore (Petryna 2007).

Welcoming foreign research also brings certain advantages to the host country: local investigators gain training and experience, clinical work is monitored with more efficiency, and a research protocol may be the only therapeutic possibility for subjects to access otherwise unavailable medication. But these fringe benefits are far from compensating the lack of privileged access to the drug being investigated.

A recent study analyses 33 clinical studies carried out in Latin American nations that were approved by the FDA between 2011 and 2012. Twenty months after their approval in the U.S. only 25% were registered in the country that hosted the trials, and one-third were approved in none of the countries involved. Where available, some of these medicaments were priced at 100-900 times the average minimum salary of those nations. In addition, the authors note how 80% of these drugs had no medical advantage over existing products. The results seem to confirm that the availability of "me too" drugs is irrelevant to people's health, but they also show that offshoring puts vulnerable subjects at unnecessary and uncompensated risks (Homedes and Ugalde 2015).

# XI. DOUBLE STANDARD IN RESEARCH ETHICS

As the tendency towards offshoring expanded, powerful sponsors and CROs became aware that certain injurious practices –sloppy informed consents, the use of placebos in control groups, the nondisclosure of research-induced harm, and the inclusion of small children and incompetent human beings in non-therapeutic trials–, would lead to litigation and costly compensations in societies with high regard for individual rights and privacy. In less-developed host countries, belatedly formed ethics committees had as yet limited experience and were presumably susceptible to lobbying and shady incentives. Sponsors and researchers argued that absolute ethical principles had to be context sensitive and give way to relative approaches adapted to local realities and idiosyncrasies, thus justifying a double standard in research ethics: an "aspirational" level of ethical excellency required in highly developed societies, and a "pragmatic" ethics adapted to low-income populations (Macklin 2004).

Should the control arm of an RCT –randomized clinical trial– receive an inert placebo or the best treatment demonstrated to be effective in comparison to the new drug being researched? Many have claimed that "best existent treatment" –aspirational ethics– should be replaced by "best

*Strategies of Biomedical Research* 69

available treatment" –pragmatic ethics–, making it ethically correct to use placebos in poor countries that lack healthcare policies and have an extremely low number of available medicines. These issues were hotly debated in HIV studies of sub-optimal treatments, and in placebo controlled trials of surfactant studies with a therapeutic agent already demonstrated to be effectively lifesaving. Comments on a trial to be carried out in Bolivia under conditions that had not been approved in a developed country, state: "The proposed Surfaxin study would therefore have been a landmark of unethical behavior –a turning to the developing world to conduct studies that the FDA acknowledged could never occur in the United States (Lurie and Wolfe 2007).

This is a prime example of the double ethical research standard: research with placebos is unacceptable to aspirational ethics in developed nations, whereas it is customary to use control groups with inactive placebos in poor host countries overseen by pragmatic ethical standards. Without going into the complexities of research ethics, the existence of a double ethical standard also impacts on availability and accessibility underlying the crucial and unresolved issue of research subjects' entitlement to the post-trial medical benefits they helped to investigate, a matter that the pharmaceutical industry claims is too costly for them to provide.

Discrimination affecting ethical research standards is by no means merely an exercise in rhetoric, for there have been proven practical consequences that were detrimental, injurious, and even lethal to underprivileged research subjects. Some clinical trials were at a stage where risks could not be predicted and benefits were uncertain, preferably carried out in less litigious communities than those at home: "The failure to predict safety outcomes or a 'paradigm of expected failure' is being exported along with the offshored clinical trial model" (Petryna 2007, 24).

Combining the effects of pragmatic research ethics, the 10/90 resources gap, outsourcing and offshoring have allowed practices that are offensively oblivious to the possible benefits for host countries and research subjects.

*Chapter 4*

# NEGLECTED AND RARE DISEASES

## I. ETHICAL MEANING OF NEGLECT

To neglect means to leave out and undone, or fail to attend to, something that requires action, omission, or non-action. Neglect needs to be evaluated as to the greater or lesser consequences it may have. To say that someone neglected to clean the windows of her home is not comparable to having neglected to feed the birds, or to neglect taking care of an aging grandmother. It is simpler to disambiguate the ethics of neglect by looking at its possible antonyms.

Neglect is not negated by its antonyms –to mind, attend to, remember, bear in mind-, nor is it adequately replaced by similar expressions –feel concern about, take responsibility, recall, bring to mind, be aware–. Neglect is not forgetfulness, or unconcern or abandonment; it is not omission –voluntary or unintended– or mere ignorance. Ignorance, even if intended, does not go beyond lack of knowledge (Latin *ignorantem*—"not knowing") and may be free of ethical connotation, whereas neglect is the failure to apply available agency towards avoiding harm or providing needed assistance. Neglect is always a moral disvalue.

Literature on nursing practices and geriatric research frequently dwell on the self-neglect of the elderly: "The inability (intentional or non-intentional) to maintain a socially and culturally accepted standard of self-care with the potential for serious consequences to the health and well-being of the self-neglecters and perhaps even to their community" (Day and Lehay-Warren 2008, 26). Self-neglect of the aged is mostly due to mental health disorders and calls for active, paternalistic intervention in tune with the nursing profession's commitment to the ethics of care. Owing to the morally negative implications of neglect, it might be more accurate to speak of the elderly's lack of self-care, which is strongly influenced by social neglect of the aging. This change of nomenclature should also help to redirect healthcare obligations away from self-responsibility and back to the public health realm.

Except for self-inflicted neglect that has no consequences for others – failing to renew one's wardrobe–, neglect is always a disvalue that harms or indolently tolerates harm that ought to and can be mitigated. The ethical significance of neglect lies with the agent who fails to account for not shaking off indifference and assuaging harm that increases if abandoned by inaction. Moral failure is the neglect or omission of expected or required action, that is, neglect occurs when agents who have the duty and power to avoid damage or suffering do not deliver. Agents ought to take responsibility and account for refraining to give the assistance that they are capable, and often under obligation, of providing. The philosophically debated distinction between acts and omissions is of little relevance in neglect issues: to omit assistance where help is due and possible has similar deleterious effects to actively diverting action elsewhere than to the neglected needy – by high-pricing essential drugs or promoting research for profit reasons–. Unrecognized misfortunes speak of insensitivity, distraction or unconcern, which may all be deplorable attitudes but do not constitute neglect in terms of failure to care or provide assistance. Neglect is guilty unresponsiveness that goes beyond failing to aid, it becomes accountable for increasing harm, therefore violating the most basic of ethical mandates, the Hippocratic *primum non nocere*, engraved in medical ethics but universally accepted as the basis of morality focused on avoiding evil or harm.

# Neglected and Rare Diseases

Responsibility is a universal ethical feature of human beings, but this does not mean that everybody is responsible for everything that occurs in the world, though many people have interpreted Sartre's demand for responsibility for all that occurs in one's own world. Diluting responsibility beyond each person's habitual realm of decision and action is unrealistic, submerging in anonymity and inactivity those who are directly responsible. Holistic views tend to create universal feelings of guilt and responsibility, and there are proposals, notably by Peter Singer, that every citizen ought to combat evil befalling the distant and unidentified (see Chapter 7-VI).

Widely comprehensive discourses often contain self-contradictions. In "her first major address" the WHO's director general Margaret Chan claimed that "Today there is no shortage of high-quality research into tropical diseases", only to add that "Low returns on investment have discouraged drug companies from allocating resources to tackle these diseases", lamenting "how academic culture that rewards publication and wealth creation...has exacerbated the problem and widened the 'translational gap'" (O'Connell 2007, 157).

## II. NEGLECT IN HEALTHCARE CONTEXTS

Neglected diseases constitute a multi-faceted reality including poverty, injustice, healthcare inequities, human rights violations, and exploitation, where multiple proximal and distal causes are involved, making it impossible to untangle their mutual interaction; the poor are vulnerable to diseases and bad health leads to poverty, just as better income improves sanitary conditions and vice versa.

An undated, unsigned web site, apparently originated from the American National Institutes of Health, and entitled "Neglected Diseases" states:

> Neglected diseases are conditions that inflict severe health burdens on the world's poorest people.

# 74                         *Miguel Kottow*

Diseases are said to be neglected if they are often overlooked by drug developers or by others instrumental in drug access, such as government officials, public health programs and the news media. Typically, private pharmaceutical companies cannot recover the cost of developing and producing treatments for these diseases.

Neglected diseases also lack visibility because they usually do not cause dramatic outbreaks that kill large numbers of people.

Further enlightenment is reached by clarifying that diseases "overlooked" and lacking "visibility" are "not considered high priorities... because they usually do not affect people who live in the United States and other developed countries" (http://rarediseases.info.nih.gov/files/neglected_Diseases_FAQs.pdf. Accessed June 20, 2018).

Multiple sources confirm the WHO's estimate that one billion people in 149 countries suffer from "one or more neglected diseases". Hardly an order of magnitude to lack visibility, be overlooked or sidetracked into anything less than high priority only because it affects others rather than developed countries.

The term "neglected diseases" is so deeply enmeshed in modern health and public health jargon that its ambiguity allows for a variety of meanings serving diverse and often contradictory purposes. The National Institute of Health (NIH) suggests that neglected diseases "are conditions that inflict severe health burdens on the world's poorest." The Pan American Health Organization (PAHO) prefers to explain that certain diseases are

Called "neglected" because of their association with the social determinant of health, inadequate access to health services, education, safe water and basic sanitation, and do not receive enough attention even though most of these diseases are treatable and can be cured with medication that costs less than one dollar.

The specialized journal *PLOS Neglected Tropical Diseases* states:

NTDs are defined as a group of poverty-promoting chronic infectious diseases, which primarily occur in rural areas and poor urban areas of

*Neglected and Rare Diseases* 75

low-income and middle-income countries. They are poverty promoting because of their impact on child health and development, pregnancy, and worker productivity, as well as their stigmatizing features.

An updated WHO report on neglected diseases describes them as "those disease understood to be primarily affecting people living in poverty in developing countries, in particular in rural areas" (Hunt 2007). Repeatedly, the WHO (2009) has described the common characteristics that "many" neglected diseases share:

- They typically affect neglected –poor, marginalized– populations.
- Their burdens can be reduced by basic public health measures.
- Existing curative measures fail to be timely available for affected populations.
- "Fear and stigma attach to some diseases, and lead to delay in seeking treatment as well as discrimination against those affected."
- Eradication and elimination of diseases may be achieved at low cost, but the cost at the national level can be significant.
- "The development of new tools –new diagnostics, drugs and vaccines– has been under-funded or neglected, largely because there has been little or no market incentive."

The fourth bullet has an undertone of blaming the victim, which should hardly, if ever, be the cause of neglect. The last item is also transcribed verbatim since it points a finger, and rightly so, at the pharmaceutical industry's persistence in market-orientated policies that are a major cause of undiminished neglect and a lack of concern for rare diseases (Mackey et al. 2014, 953–954).

Many sources prefer to simply list the neglected tropical diseases, and refer to them as a diverse group of about 17 to 20 tropical infections occurring in low-income populations of Africa, Asia and the Americas – notably Central America and the Northern part of South America–. The denomination of neglected diseases is neither static nor uniformly specified, and has required reshuffling as emerging infectious diseases (EIDs) and re-emerging (REIDs) ones, drawing concerned attention mostly because of changes in causal mechanisms and altered dissemination factors that threaten rich and poor.

These conceptual vagaries make neglected diseases a boundary object, that is, a reality that is diversely seen in the light of different perspectives, thus receiving a variety of meanings. Neglected diseases may be seen as an instance of wide socioeconomic disparity between rich and poor, as a political problem subject to the exercise of power, as a matter of scientific policies that set their own priorities. There are many pathways to neglect, which need to be singled out in order to place responsibilities and evaluate improvement policies.

The term neglected diseases is just a specific way of referring to the more comprehensive concept of neglected populations, though this would reinforce the viewpoint that we are facing a holistic situation requiring global responses, which the entrenched and increasing negativities of socioeconomic disparities are turning into bundles of unassailable and irreversible harm. Alternative credence is given to the belief that the destitute are architects of their own fate, their misery not being man-made but due to unfortunate moral luck, a train of thought shortsightedly indulging in a rhetoric that fits snuggly into neoliberal equal opportunity doctrine and to the proclamation that all human beings are born equal in dignity and rights.

A good reason for approaching the subject in a more differentiated way than juggling attractive but unfeasible ideas like human solidarity, cosmopolitan parliaments, universal values, or other holistic values, is to accept that huge problems are invariably downsized to specified focal solutions, as often suggested by ecologists and communal theorists: "think global, act local." For the subject of neglected diseases, global thinking is needed for a comprehensive understanding of the problem together with the search for realistic therapeutic strategies expected to "act local and focal".

# III. POVERTY AND NEGLECT

The first issue of *PLOS Neglected Tropical Diseases* carried an editorial with the title "A New Voice for the Poor" (Hotez 2007, 1), setting the pace to address tropical infectious diseases, that affected the poor population, mostly but not exclusively in low-income nations.

The majority of people are not aware that "the share of extremely poor people has fallen faster than ever before in history over the last 30 years"; in fact, the common impression is that poverty has increased. The discrepancy is probably due to the fact that World Bank criteria are not relevant to daily life experience, where the general population is seeing a decline of purchasing power as prices rise and incomes decline or stagnate. Citizens of the Western world are supposedly gaining in autonomy but losing in social protection as they live in uncertainty and insecurity, raising the suspicion that socioeconomic development is mainly favorable to the privileged, while statistics show that the poor are merely hovering above the $2.00 income per day threshold. These meager rises are barely significant in terms of empowerment and perspectives to rise from the destitution of extreme poverty to the neediness of the relative poor who continue to be victims of neglected diseases living in low-income countries, and in pockets of destitution in richer nations.

Crossing lines from extreme poverty to low-income poverty, and from here to middle-income conditions, fails to distinguish between absolute poverty –the incapacity to acquire basic survival goods–, and relative poverty –low income that is 50% less than the median income–. Income-based determinations of poverty need to be contextualized for nations that provide social sustenance, and those where no kind of income subsidy and social protection is available. A more realistic approach has been presented as "multidimensional poverty" which includes evaluating health –nutrition and child mortality–, education, and living standards –water, sanitation, habitat, and energy– (Alkire and Foster 2008). The formula for measuring poverty is the MPI (Multidimensional poverty index) = H (incidence) x A (intensity), a calculus based on available data, for the purpose of designing effective, coherent policies. The question remains whether quantitative approaches will have the pull to motivate a comprehensive focus on reducing world poverty, unless an ethical motivation becomes culturally ingrained to pursue goals of fairness.

Poverty and inequity are problems of global concern, but none other than the United Nations Bill of Rights –the Declaration plus Covenants– has defused global action to deal with socioeconomic disparity and its dire consequences for basic biological needs including healthcare: firstly, it has supported a policy of "progressive realization" (see Chapter 7-II) and; secondly, it has repeatedly made it clear that solutions are up to the resources and strength of each nation: the 1966 International Covenant on Civil and Political Rights states in its "Preamble": "Considering the obligation of States under the Charter of the United Nations to promote universal respect for, and observance of, human rights and freedoms."

The multiple global initiatives presented by the WHO offer an international deliberation forum which provides laundry lists that individual States are encouraged to consider to the best of their ability and resources. "A right to health-related goods is compatible with the unfortunate likelihood that it will not be honored for the majority of the world's poor for many years to come" (Arras and Fenton 2009, 32).

"Think global, act local", traps the needy in the vicious circle of poor countries being unable to improve their government's solvency to attend and relieve the problems of its destitute population, unless high and high-middle income countries shake off their indolence to assist the underprivileged to reach at least a minimum of welfare. As matters stand, humanitarian views based on rights are helplessly unable to get a foothold in world affairs that have bowed to the instrumental force of neoliberalism's polarization of inequities.

> The institution [World Bank] became an integral part of the so-called 'Washington consensus' that imposed harsh conditions on lending and repayment on many countries, conditions that interfered more and more with their ability to engage in state provision. (Moyn 2018, 190)

*Neglected and Rare Diseases*                79

The enormous power and resilience of social and economic forces are reflected in what John Galtung has studied as the "triangle of violence" including direct, structural and cultural violence. Paul Farmer, a physician and anthropologist with vast firsthand experience in providing medical care in poor countries, writes about structural violence directly connected to poverty, human rights violation and disease (Farmer 2003). His experience tells him that structural violence transgresses human rights, exacerbating poverty and its sequels, notably disease and reduced life expectancy, a chain of processes that he sees as pathologies of power. Poverty caused disease, and disease intensified poverty, thus explaining why one billion of the poorest harbor one or more NTDs, caught in the vicious circle of unmitigated misery.

Farmer's perceptive writings refer to political regimes and restrictive migration policies that violate human rights to the point of creating situations of disease, suffering and death. This repressive form of power needs to be eliminated, but neglect is more a matter of guilty indifference than aggressive violence, hardly mitigated by proclaiming respect for human rights without acting to support them. Neglected people, unable to come to the starting line of equal opportunities will not be helped by touting individual autonomy unaccompanied by empowerment, without seriously addressing the prevalent and increasing disparity of income and of basic social needs like healthcare and education.

Power is not only repressive it is exerted by the stick but also by the word. Democratic societies exert power through a pretense of truth and unmet promises of material fairness, shifting from questions about who holds power to questions about forms and operations of power that "categorize the individual, mark him by his own individuality, attach him to his own identity, impose a law of truth on him which he must recognize and which others must recognize in him... a form of power which makes individuals subjects" as Foucault wrote in 1982 (Brown 2006, 67). Further discussing this Foucauldian idea, Brown confirms that "discourses of health, consumerism, or safety are as or more important than discourses of rights in governing the contemporary liberal democratic subject" (Ibid., 74).

The job of unveiling the miseries caused by inequity has been meticulously done, in fact overdone, because too much exposure leads to fatigue and insensitivity, finally returning neglect to the basket of neglected issues. Waiting for progressive realization without specifying commitment as to timespan for goals to be attained, condemns the marginalized to stagnate in the cesspool of neglect.

Embedded in the dominant and unassailable socioeconomic conditions of our times, concern about neglect must begin by modestly searching for its way through the more proximal causes that carry their own momentum in the carnival of market fundamentalism.

Public health policies try to identify distant and proximal causes of disease, the latter being more amenable to diagnostic recognition and effective treatment of immediate disease-triggering situations. Prevalent tuberculosis is treated with appropriate antibiotics and supportive measures, though the association of poor living conditions with the incidence and severity of this disease is well known. Tuberculosis is by and large amenable to medical treatment and public health policies, but also presents as a re-emergent drug-resistant condition showing that proximal treatment alone without attacking distant conditions will provide only temporary relief. Similar considerations pertain to non-infectious chronic diseases where the main causal culprit is said to be lifestyle, but partially effective therapies are often necessarily directed at proximal causes by using anti-hypertensive drugs, statins, bariatric surgery for obesity, and anti-ageing medication for the elderly. If structural pathogenicity is not changed, biomedical treatment will continue to provide inefficient and costly medicalization that benefits providers more than it alleviates suffering from chronic disease. Medical sociology has often remarked that the chronically ill, as the aged, are subjected to medicalization in a social milieu of neglected care.

Structural globalized conditions are bemoaned but unchanged, while healthcare measures are steeped in inequality and neglect of the underprivileged. Neglect is widespread, pervasive and unassailable, suggesting the need to act focally despite its short-term effects, that is,

# Neglected and Rare Diseases

exacting where and by what acts or omissions diseases are being unattended to the point of neglect that can no longer be tolerated.

Recent updates by the Center for Disease Control and Prevention (CDC) claim that six neglected tropical diseases can be controlled by using "mass drug administration" (MDA) and other effective tools that make these diseases "targeted" or "tool ready". And yet, they continue to be listed among the neglected diseases. Always hidden, NTDs became increasingly submerged in invisibility as massive efforts were being developed to combat the three major killers also called the "big three" – HIV/AIDS, tuberculosis and malaria–.

Along with MDA and direct interventions, we are told, efforts to control the vectors (e.g., mosquitoes, black flies) that transmit these diseases, and to improve basic water, sanitation, and hygiene, are highly effective strategies against these NTDs. If such programs are actually being implemented, the disease in this group should no longer be seen as neglected. Reports and reviews are difficult to interpret, celebrating improvements at the same time that they issue *caveats*: research will be necessary, coverage and adherence are inadequate, progress has been patchy. The often repeated, and stubbornly valid, definition of NTDs as a "group of infections strongly associated with poverty in tropical and subtropical environments" (Molyneux, Savoli, Engels 2017, 312), can be read as questioning the statement "During the past decade, NTDs have attracted increased attention and investment" (Ibid., 322).

Scientific reports on prevalence, effective treatment, focalized R&D, financial support, availability, accessibility, and favorable epidemiological reports, are all presented in arrays of numbers and statistics that may lead to diverse conclusions. A Global Burden disease study (2010) places the number of disability adjusted life years (DALYs) attributed to NTDS at 27 million, whereas another study (2014) comes up with 47.9 million DALYs, and a third one (2009) refers to 56 million. If the results were comparable, which they are not since the number of diseases included varies, they would show things to be getting worse over a period of 5 years, illustrating how the prosperous and privileged show little interest in, and responsibility for, the misery and suffering of the destitute.

Other parameters like accessibility and supportive public health measures are even less quantifiable. A major cause of persistent health neglect is the lack of motivation in developing preventive and therapeutic agents that the needy require but are unable to pay for, thus confirming that neglected and rare diseases are really those that have low priority in R&D. The indifference and downright opposition to devoting more resources and scientific efforts to diseases having low R&D priority have powerful financial causes exacerbated by structural conditions that erect firm obstacles against change.

> The current system for the research and development (R&D) of new medicines does not adequately meet the needs of the majority of the world's population…, over 80% of which live in low and middle-income countries. (We use the general term 'medicines' to refer broadly to drugs, vaccines, diagnostics, and other medical products.) (Moon, Berez, t´Hoen 2012, 1).

## IV. EMERGENT AND RE-EMERGENT INFECTIOUS DISEASES (EIDS AND REIDS)

Much concern comes from the U.S. Center for Disease Control and Prevention (CDC) focused on infections that are increasing over time or threaten to do so, adding "new infections resulting from new unknown pathogens, known infections which are increasing over new geographic areas, and known infections that are re-emerging as a result of both resistance to antimicrobial therapies and the failure of public health measures" (Mackey et al. 2014, 951). The U.S. National Institutes of Health (NIH) classify emerging and re-emerging into three groups, subdividing Group 3 into categories A, B and C according to "potential bioterrorism threats": "Category A priority, poses highest risk to national security and public health, easily disseminated/high mortality" –including poxviruses, anthrax, and botulism–; "Category B priority, second-highest priority, moderately easy to disseminate/low mortality" –typhus fever, food

# Neglected and Rare Diseases

and waterborne pathogens–; "Category C, third-highest priority, includes emerging pathogens that could be mass produced and easily disseminated" –rabies, influenza, and hanta viruses–.

These and other lists of EIDs and REIDs are part of the NTDs – EReNTD– that admit flexible modifications, as occurred with the 2017 WHO inclusion of snakebite envenoming, which is a non-infectious, serious and often lethal accident, of high incidence in tropical areas, where poor people often lack protective footwear, and are isolated from healthcare facilities where prompt treatment with antivenom agents is crucial. Furthermore, the CDC's emphasis on "potential bioterrorism threats" reveals a shift of emphasis from assistance to defence, and from poverty to security, that is bound to modify strategies, resource allocations and R&D preferences going beyond the realm of NTDs. Diseases may be distant but if the privileged feel threatened, they will trigger massive responses, as shown by the intensive research to limit the worldwide spreading of HIV that respects no social barriers. Interest in anthrax, smallpox and other viruses is heightened by the fear of biological terrorist attacks, way beyond concern for the endemic conditions that affect the poor, like faraway sleeping sickness or Chagas disease.

## V. BLUE MARBLE DISEASE

By 2013, the WHO was applying DALY metrics (Disability Adjusted Life Year) to calculate the global burden of disease –GBD–, estimating that about half of many NTDs also affect the poor living in wealthy countries, a fact that had remained unnoticed because neglected diseases have a relatively low mortality but very high morbidity resulting in many years of disablement, disfigurement and chronic ailment. The catastrophic global health conditions triggered the search for low-cost "rapid impact packages" of essential medicines and mass drug administration known as "preventive chemotherapy", but again, the impact of these policies was weakened by unattended structural problems.

The G20 nations plus Nigeria, were dubbed the "blue marble health countries", a name reminiscent of the 1972 photographic image of the Earth produced by an Apollo mission, signaling the health needs of the poorer segments of wealthy economies suffering from NTDs. A major shift in combatting NTDs required these nations to take "greater ownership of their own public health control and policy efforts" to "eliminate at last one-half of the world's neglected diseases (Hotez, Damania and Naghavi 2016, 1).

Neglected people may live in communities that may have an agenda of improving their lot on their own terms, that is, according to their internal values and hopes, and will gladly adopt external assistance provided their culture and morals are respected. Yet, they do not conform to an organized social movement to which activists may adhere. Combating discrimination and advocating recognition of the distant needy require the dissolving of ingrained attitudes that are unaware of or indifferent to the harm they cause.

Giving credit where credit is due, leprosy has been drastically reduced in many countries (116/122), as well as dracunculiasis, onchocerciasis and the incidence and severity of a number of other NTDs in certain regions of endemicity. These programs have been made possible in part due to medicine donations (primarily in the form of preventive chemotherapy from a number of [major] pharmaceutical manufacturers. Drug-based medication and vaccines have at times been generously supported by the U.S., Britain, and by wealthy foundations like the Bill and Melinda Gates Foundation. These efforts in treating and preventing NTDs are to be acknowledged in their impact on caring for the sick and reducing the incidence of many endemic diseases.

Equally admirable is the program, Drugs for Neglected Diseases Initiative (DNDI), where Médecins Sans Frontières plays a major role in sustaining non-profit drug research and development (R&D) of new treatments for neglected diseases. Operating since 2003, the organization has efficiently improved access to existing drugs and developed entirely new chemical entities, delivering healthcare according to local needs and participation. Furthermore, the pharmaceutical industry's occasional

## Neglected and Rare Diseases

generous supply of drugs and vaccines for neglected diseases is a humanitarian aid that contrasts sharply with their profit-oriented strategies that have extremely negative effects on the development and availability of their products.

And yet, these laudable endeavors are often criticized for keeping poor populations enclosed in their hopeless situations, vulnerable to other emerging and re-emerging diseases, to drug-resistant reinfections, and trapped in chronic suffering, as is to be expected when assistance is only weakly or not at all accompanied by empowerment and structural changes. Once again, assistance without empowerment results in only temporary relief as long as structures of power are not changed.

These are other concerns that touch on the issue of neglected diseases: international money loans to the LMIC are conditioned to privatization in many areas, notably in medical care and public health policies.

> Captured by the slogan 'Trade Not Aid', the ethical imperative of reducing aid-dependency is increasingly supported by well-intended voices from the so-called 'global South' as well as from the 'global North'…We also support efforts to make international trade 'fairer'. However, we do not understand why both claims are linked and treated as mutually exclusive: why 'trade, not aid' instead of 'trade and aid'? (Ooms and Hammonds 2008, 154)

In 2010, a Consultative Expert Working Group (CEWG) was established to analyze, plan and recommend actions and policies to face the threats of NTDs. Funding for global R&D was found to be product inadequate, product development was sparse owing to insufficient incentives for private-sector investment, and there were deficiencies in current intellectual property systems. The promotion of "true" public-private partnerships needs to be encouraged, as well as aiming at

> A new level of regulatory science required with a need for capacity building among many national regulatory countries in low and middle-income countries, as well as capacity building for research institutions in

86                                  *Miguel Kottow*

disease-endemic countries to partner with developing country manufacturers. (Hotez 2013, 3)

The richness and variety of proposals to deal with NTDs lead to the conclusion that these global health problems are no longer neglected through invisibility, but rather through the lack of audacious, imaginative and clearly oriented action. Funding is chronically insufficient and decreasing, but this is hardly the main and sufficient reason for failure: "Reliance solely on perpetual philanthropy is clearly not the long-term answer to global health problems" (Benatar 2005, 1209). Many problems are due to the absence of integration and innovation, and the persistence of negative social factors –civil strife, unstable local communities–. The ecological problems surrounding tropical diseases have prompted convergence with the Sustainable Development Goals, sharing their aim but also their problems (see Chapter 1-V). Some major initiatives are, or have been, engaged in tackling the NTD problems: One Health –uniting medical and veterinarian programs–, the Global Fund –initially focused on HIV, tuberculosis and malaria, later expanding to included NTDs–, and some prize funds.

Emergence and re-emergence of old and new infectious diseases alike continue worldwide, are complex and multidisciplinary, involve a host of contributing factors, and are now accelerated by globalization, presenting unique challenges for collective global public health efforts and health security. At the same time, neglected tropical diseases continue to be a blight on human progress and remain critical impediments to alleviate worldwide poverty as envisioned by the international community through the MDGs.

Though scientific progress in addressing some infectious diseases is moving forward, the goals of elimination and eradication of all NTDs remain largely distant. Within this context, EReNTDs represent a subset of infectious disease that require close attention. These diseases have the potential to emerge/re-emerge while remaining neglected in the global health priority. (Mackey et al. 2014, 969)

*Neglected and Rare Diseases* 87

In a 2017 report the WHO states: "Although only 4.1% of new and 19% of retreatment TB cases have MDR/RR-TB, globally they amount to ~600,000 incident cases each year, challenging the prospect of ending TB by 2035." Global HIV prevention targets continue to be missed by a wide margin and declines in new HIV infections remain too slow. Tellingly, only 2.1 million (6%) people living with HIV live in Western and Central Europe and North America.

Exploring the social topography of neglected tropical diseases unveils some landmarks that will continue to reshape this basic reality of health/disease issues in the modern world. Neglected diseases are no longer exclusively tropical, as they become a worldwide scourge. Nor are they mainly infectious, since chronicity, complications, sequels and disabilities require more comprehensive healthcare than only medicating or preventing an acute infection. Chagas disease, for example, is an acute infection that causes systemic pathology in its chronic phase –heart disease, intestinal problems, and central nervous system involvement–. The enormous worldwide spread of dengue infections is threatening poor and not so poor populations affected by non-transmissible chronic diseases (NCDs) like diabetes and hypertension, causing more severe cases of dengue, as well as complicated and often lethal co-morbidities: "Dengue and its co-morbidities represent an important example of the overlap between NTDs and NCDs, especially among the poor" (Metha and Hotez 2016, 3). Initial but mounting evidence indicates a mutual exacerbation between dengue and NCDs.

The major thrust against neglected diseases is based on therapeutic and preventive substances –drugs and vaccines–. Public health measures against neglected diseases are proximal or downstream –biological–, yet their underlying causes –socioeconomic determinants– are distal or upstream. Proximal/distal causality is often employed in public health debates, creating what some scholars, notably Nancy Krieger, consider an artificial and confusing separation of conjoint causalities. Actions to combat NTD are mostly based on direct technical intervention –therapeutic medication and preventive vaccination– based on a proximal approach, which in the long run may have only transient effects considering that the basic upstream causes of poverty, inequity and disempowerment will continue to heavily maintain the global burden of NTDs. These *de facto* separations between what is technically possible and what is politically, socially and economically necessary, debunk a more comprehensive and effective approach to eradicating neglect in healthcare matters.

Many aspects of preventing, treating, controlling and eliminating NTDs need to be developed and perfected to resolve the main obstacles that hinder and delay reaching these goals. Worldwide globalization is in full swing and will most probably not change its course in the foreseeable future; low-income countries and the poor populations in these and also in wealthier nations will continue to be trapped under the negative influence of socioeconomic factors that lead to an unfair distribution of goods and services and mounting healthcare disparities, nursed by weakened governments unable to provide basic social security. Extreme poverty is declining in terms of income, which does not necessarily increase the purchasing power of the poor, or help to improve access to healthcare facilities.

> Technologies such as vaccines and antiretroviral drugs have the potential to deliver a generational leap in achieving the Millennium Development Goals. The health gains made in Europe in the past 150 years could be achieved in Africa within the next 10 to 20 years. But without an accelerated and coordinated effort to tackle the fundamental constraint –weak infrastructure for the delivery of basic health care– the full potential of innovative strategies will not be realized. (Affolder et al. 2007, 172)

## VI. BRAZIL AND TEXAS: CASE STUDIES

Two blue marble health areas arise where the high prevalence of NTDs is barely acknowledged and persistently unheeded –Texas–; and where the pertinent healthcare measures in Brazil are dismantled at the most probable risk that the incidence of NTDs will drastically increase. In any case, blue

*Neglected and Rare Diseases* 89

marble health areas riddled with NTDs are not up to the task of moving from neglect to concerned attention and effective measures to control these sanitary problems, constituting a discouraging omen for counteracting NTDs in poor countries and populations trapped in poverty.

The US Gulf Coast states harbor an alarming rate of poor populations approximating 10 million people who live below the poverty line. "Severe poverty, climate changes and warming, human migrations and changing patterns of global shipping produce a 'perfect storm' for ongoing NTD transmission on the Gulf Coast" (Hotez and Lee 2017, 3). The prevalence and incidence of parasitic and vector-borne diseases are estimated to be high and, on the rise and the increased risk of Zika virus has not received timely priority by the US Government. The at-risk population living on the Gulf is seen as the "'flyover nation'… ignored by a government and media biased in favour of urban centers in the Northeast, Southeastern California, or Silicon Valley" (Ibid., 1).

> 'New' Texas [is] beset by modern and globalizing forces that include rapid expansions in population together with urbanization and human migrations, altered transportation patterns, climate change, steeply declining vaccination rates, and a new paradigm of poverty, known as 'blue marble death'. (Hotez 2018, 1)

The state of Texas has been singled out as a prime example of blue marble health conditions. Growing and exceedingly urbanized, Texas is one of the wealthiest states in the U.S., ranking "among the states with the largest number of people living in poverty of any US state land near the bottom (41st) in terms of food insecurity and educational attainment" (Ibid., 2). The region is plagued by climate change and at disproportionate risk of global warming, and ecological deterioration. Preliminary data show a widespread prevalence of vector-borne NTDs –West Nile Virus, Chagas disease, typhus, zoonotic helminth infections, and protozoan and sexually transmitted NTDs–. Public measures, including improved diagnostics, efficient and accessible drugs and vaccines are insufficient and, unless housing, sanitation, and access to healthcare are significantly improved, "the prevalence and incidence of NTDs could increase in the coming years" (Ibid., 10).

Though plagued in recent years by political instability, fiscal scandals and a stalling economy, Brazil is a member of the rapidly expanding economies, together with Russia India and China –the BRIC countries–, and also included in the G20 group of the world's strongest economies. Over the last two decades, Brazil has reduced its poverty rates, created the SUS –Servicio Único de Saúde (national healthcare service)–, improved its healthcare indicators and successfully reduced endemic malaria. Healthcare reforms and policies were overambitious and did not live up to expectations, but the Brazilian population obtained significant improvements in medical care and public health protection.

In the wake of a weakened economy, Brazil introduced in 2016-17 severe budget cuts leading to austerity, privatization, and deregulation. Federal budgets including health spending were frozen, health-related sectors –education and science– suffered major cuts, and social protection plans were reduced or cancelled. Commercial health plans and privatized healthcare replaced the free SUS services and increased out-of-pocket expenditures. Federal public health measures were regionalized thus increasing geographic health inequalities: "The weakening of the public sector has also taken a toll on vaccination coverage and sanitary surveillance, resulting in a recent outbreak of measles" (Doniec, Dall'Alba and King 2018, 731).

# VII. RARE DISEASES

Rare diseases are a specific group of diseases that are mostly, but not all, extremely infrequent, being inefficiently researched, while coming up with very high-priced therapeutic agents –amyotrophic lateral sclerosis, multiple sclerosis, T-cell lymphoma, and pheochromocytoma–. Many up-coming drugs share three characteristics that make them unaffordable: a high price, an insufficiently subsidized out-of-pocket expense, and

# Neglected and Rare Diseases

palliative rather than curative effects that require long-term, even life-long treatment.

Even though about 35-40 million persons are affected by genetically determined rare diseases statistics have been unable to recruit research funds to accelerate scientific programs aimed at effective mitigation, retardation, symptomatic relief or improved functionality for affected patients. Most efforts are centered on the study of genetic anomalies and prenatal detection that is of little use if the abortion laws are too restrictive to allow the voluntary abortion of unborn embryos or fetuses condemned to what Hobbes described, in a different context, as a solitary, poor, nasty, brutish and short life, steeped in medical life-salvaging efforts, with disrupting consequences for family life and the commitment of care-givers. Rare diseases are a matter of misdirected biomedical research efforts.

Being of genetic origin, most rare diseases largely affect children. Some of the more developed countries –foremost the European Union– are creating awareness and implementing programs to offer specialized pediatric medical care and social services in an effort to alleviate the heavy disease burden of patients and their families. Countries with emerging and low-income economies, which have higher birth rates and therefore a higher incidence of rare diseases, are yet far away from being able to provide these services, confirming once more the disparities of healthcare between the wealthy and the disadvantaged (Bavisetty, Grody and Yazdani 2013).

A review of Huntington's disease can be applied to the majority of rare diseases: "To date, despite several claims, no drug is available with any neuroprotective or disease-delaying effect. Disease modifying drugs are developed, but not available. Also embryonic cell implants, still under study, are not proven treatment options at the moment" (Roos 2010).

There are great similarities between neglected and rare diseases. In fact, rare diseases are a sub-group of neglected ailments, but they follow their own specific dynamics of abandonment and neglect. Rare diseases used to be a vague medical concept reminding physicians to keep in mind that they might encounter some very infrequent clinical pictures or atypical and misleading presentations of an otherwise familiar disease. The concept

92                                   *Miguel Kottow*

became current in the mid-1970s in the *Orphan Drug Act* (U.S. 1984), enacted in the wake of the requirement to demonstrate the efficacy of current pharmaceutical products.

The need to regulate the use and prescription of drugs was triggered by the thalidomide tragedy. A German pharmaceutical company had registered and launched a non-barbiturate tranquilizer guaranteed to be so safe that it could be sold over the counter, that is, without a medical prescription. An off-label indication as a remedy for morning sickness increased the use of thalidomide up till 1962, when thousands of children with malformed or even absent extremities –phocomelia– were born, all cases occurring where thalidomide had been used within the first trimester of pregnancy. In the U.S., FDA scientist Frances O. Kelsey delayed approval of the drug, posing that its safety in pregnant women had not been satisfactorily demonstrated. This fortunate stand averted the use of thalidomide, triggering the Kefauver-Harris amendment to the Food, Drug and Cosmetic Act regarding drugs in current use, where companies should prove the effectiveness of their products or withdraw them from the market. Some drugs were not subjected to this review process of medical usefulness, nor were they withdrawn although they had no legal authorization to be employed. Not being classified as successfully reviewed or as withdrawn, this group of drugs was "homeless" and they began to be known as orphan drugs, defined by the *Orphan Drug Act* of 1983 as "non-profitable drugs".

Orphan non-profitable drugs included drugs for uncommon diseases, causing the alarm of physicians and patients who feared that the treatment of their conditions would face increasing obstacles. "For a decade, two different issues developed into non-profitable drugs on the one hand and into drugs for rare diseases on the other."

> They merged in 1984, in the second version of the *Orphan Drug Act,* which specified that a drug for which the orphan status was solicited should either: 1) affect less than 200,000 persons in the United States of America; or 2) affect more than 200,000 persons but be unlikely to be profitable in the US. With hindsight, it appears that the second criterion

# Neglected and Rare Diseases

has never been used...so orphan drugs are drugs for rare disease. (Huyard 2013, 466)

As the National Organization for Rare Disorders –NORD– was formed, public opinion pressed for incentives that were expected to seduce the pharmaceutical world into actively researching and developing therapeutic agents for rare diseases. Incentives ran from tax exemptions to lengthy and eventually renewable marketing exclusivity, thus unwittingly but consistently supporting inordinately high-priced products.

The Therapeutics for Rare and Neglected Diseases (TRND) is a collaborative program of academic scientists and the NIH (National Institutes of Health) that aims to "encourage and speed the development of new treatments for disease with high unmet medical needs." The NIH has issued an informative text on "Neglected diseases", defining them as "conditions that inflict severe health burden on the world's poorest people", and giving as a cause for this neglect the fact that "private pharmaceutical companies cannot recover the cost of developing and producing treatments for these diseases" (https://rarediseases.info.nih.gov/files/neglected_Disease_FAWS.pdf).

The orphan condition is a category often applied to diseases that are undiagnosed by doctors because they occur infrequently. Orphanhood can apply to neurodegenerative disorders, rare forms of cancer, extremely infrequent genetic diseases, and even to NTDs waylaid by healthcare authorities and services, for the most part having in common insufficient R&D, hindered availability and prohibitive accessibility. In general, the term "rare diseases" is preferred for defining conditions of extreme low incidence, varying from 1 in 200,000 in the U.S. and less than 5 in 10,000 for the European Community. Over 6,000 rare diseases have been described, but the list is growing as exceptional forms of otherwise frequent diseases are found and genetic findings pinpoint disorders of hitherto unrecognized clinical manifestations.

Orphan drugs are employed to treat rare diseases. R&D for these drugs is technically complicated, costly and lengthy. The low prevalence hinders clinical trials from achieving significant results, discouraging researchers and sponsors from embarking on research efforts that will have low sales and unsatisfactory profits. Push/pull incentives include tax credits and research aids, simplified procedures to reach the market and, notably in Europe, extended market exclusivity (see Chapter 7).

> Currently drug companies do not have a financial incentive to invest in developing new drugs for rare or 'orphan' diseases due to the small proportion of the population who are affected and the high costs and uncertain outcomes of the drug development process. (Halpin et al. 2015, 987)

> Thirty-four years have passed since the passage of the US Orphan Drug Act. More than 500 drugs have been approved for marketing by the US Food and Drug Administration for the treatment of rare/orphan diseases. Countless numbers of patients and their families have been provided needed therapies with the assistance of the economic incentives of the program. The program has been implemented in some way in many parts of the world. Many 'cutting edge' therapies have seen their first approval as a result of the US Orphan Drug Act. (Haffner 2016, 343)

Such contradictory appraisals are abundant, illustrating the difficulties in supporting solid views on this controversy. Incentives for research on rare diseases have at times been successful both in the U.S. and in Europe, but that initial momentum has decelerated as the pharmaceutical industry decides that even subsidized research will not compensate for investment in developing non-profitable rare disease drugs. The most sought after incentive is a lengthy exclusivity period, during which drug producers exercise the market power of demanding unlimited high prices to scoop up enormous profits before competition threatens their monopoly. Secondly, it is extremely difficult to assess whether innovative therapies demonstrably help to improve the clinical status of rare disease patients. Thirdly, even effective therapies are so costly that they exceed the payment capacities of insurance and national healthcare services, leading to reticent approval and the registration of drugs that show uncertain and weak cost/effectiveness ratios. If DALY calculations are resorted to, rare diseases will mostly qualify for the short end, given that costly treatments will deliver only limited disease-free additional life-years. Rationalizing schemes for high-cost therapies has been erratic and unsatisfactory because inclusion/exclusion criteria rarely find economic and ethical consensus.

*Chapter 5*

# MEDICAL ANTHROPOLOGY FOR BIOETHICS

## I. ANTHROPOLOGY AND BIOETHICS

The interaction between anthropology and bioethics has had an irregularly flirtatious character, with the latter usually being the wooed one. Anthropology offers to enrich and give more substance to bioethics.

Anthropologists can contribute to the fields of medical ethics and bioethics in two significant ways: Of critical importance is the inherent complexity of individual and cultural values concerning the nature of illness, the management of medical care, and the use of medical technologies. (Marshall 1992, 62)

Ethics and values cannot be separated from social, cultural, and historical determinants that regulate both the definition and resolution of moral quandaries...Morality and medical practice are embedded in culture,...Warren believes bioethics needs: 'In medical ethics, we need to do a lot more listening'. (Muller 1994, 453, 459)

Fortunately, Muller acknowledges a "growing number of examples of writings by non-anthropologists who are sensitive to these issues" (Ibid., 453). Non-experts ought to be additionally welcome when concern is about the search for basic anthropological features expected to ease the way to

98                     *Miguel Kottow*

the bioethics approach to neglected disease. What follows is the use of a free ticket to browse thoughts on human nature.


## II. ANTHROPOLOGY AND THE NATURE OF THE HUMAN

Humans have invariably taken pride of place in nature and among living beings, based on the historical belief in their divine origin as creatures endowed with the rationality of *homo sapiens sapiens*, an exceptional species that dominates over all of nature. After replacing theocentric cosmology with a down-to-earth anthropocentric worldview, Western culture basks in its exceptionality at mastering self-driven cultural control over nature. Darwin's explanation of how species evolve and are not created, together with the scientific unveiling of remarkable genomic similarities between hominids and humans, has challenged this purported exceptionality of the human species. The efficacy of manipulating nature is questioned when related to the high ecological costs of depleting natural resources and polluting the world, with a pressing need to regulate human intervention in natural processes.

Well-known Darwinist Helena Cronin has repeatedly insisted that human nature is fixed, universal and unchanging, yet allows for a wide display of human behavior generated with endless variability and diversity. This is quite a statement considering that we are unable to define the human unchanging nature, philosophers despairing and mostly coming to deny that such an essential nature exists. "Appeals to human nature are, like appeals to political will, no more than graceful camouflage for disguising awkward ignorance" (Kleinman 1999, 74).

The view that nature has intrinsic value and meaning is gallantly defended by humanists but staunchly rejected by hard-core scientists. Defense of nature *per se* is not always as romantic and altruistic as one might think, arguments ranging from aesthetic pleasure to stark calls for survival of the human species.

Even though nature remains a fundamental ontological concept of reality, the borders liquefy between the physical world and humankind's development of cultures in constant tension with conservationists pulling back on expanding forces of control and intervention. The nature/culture dichotomy is disappearing as technoscience subjects natural reality to a limitless artifactual transformation. The utopia of post-humanity is finding its place in ongoing debates ranging from science to philosophy, from a grave "do not" to a lightheaded "why not?" Nanotechnology is developing the capabilities to manipulate matter at the atomic and molecular levels, and coming to create new materials and structures.

Alarmed ecologists point out that "playing God" is destroying the planet. Humanity is expected to accept that rights talk must include nonhuman living beings and respect the intrinsic value of the natural. Biodiversity in nature and dignity in the human are posed as untouchable due to their intrinsic value, rejecting that inherent worth "is a product of a particular culture and world view and a particular economic system," as presented in an August 2018 issue of *Nature* discussing "The Battle for the Soul of Biodiversity".

Anthropology, arguably initiated by Kant with the question "What is man?", has struggled with a variety of unsatisfactory answers and descriptions of the human that remain conjectural since it is impossible to revise them from an outside perspective. Cultural achievements have led philosophers like Henri Bergson to prefer the designation of *homo faber*, while others stress the primary importance of religiosity, sociality, playfulness, and a seemingly endless list, moving Heidegger to complain that, since the ontological nature of the human was unknown, humanism should refrain from labeling and thus obstructing the search for the nature of Being. Heidegger develops the existentialist stance that sees the human being as *Dasein*, a conscious and active being-in-the-world. A world that is perceived through the organic, living body that is born, matures, decays and dies.

From times immemorial, the utter finitude of the human body seemed unacceptable and was countered by hoping that some part of it would assuredly be rescued beyond death. Human beings, perhaps even animals – *pace* Descartes–, were expected to participate in a non-organic afterlife, thus sustaining the belief that the body had a finite biological life harboring a force or energy –soul, spirit– that survives beyond death.

The duality of body and soul, or mind/body, prevails as a fountain of meaning and destiny sustained by the humanities, the evolution of history and progress. Obstacles to human integrity and development are condemned as social evils of unbridled "dehumanization", occurring in dire situations varying from concentration camps to "savage capitalism", from marginalization to administered and profit-seeking medical practices, exclusion, neglect and exploitation, all of which increase the vulnerability and suffering of human bodies. Trying to distinguish between soul and body is irrelevant to the wretched who, so says Nietzsche, are placated by empty religious promises of an afterlife of redress.

The substantial distinction of soul and body is most injurious when bodily suffering receives meaning because it fortifies the spirit. C. S. Lewis tried to convince the world that pain is God's megaphone to rouse the tepid belief of a deaf world. The Book of Job can be read as asserting that the flesh is to suffer so the soul-imbued body may be redeemed. Injury to or annihilation of the body furthered by religious fanaticism in the name of a graced afterlife has caused much unnecessary human suffering and inhumane mistreatment.

Emmanuel Lévinas writes in one of his always fine-grained texts, that the suffering of others is intolerable: "For anyone ethically sensitive, justifying the suffering of my neighbor would be the scandalous origin of all immorality" (Lévinas 1991, 126). Inflicted suffering is meaningless and therefore cannot be explained, it epitomizes Hannah Arendt's banality of evil (see Chapter 9-B). Although both were reacting to the atrocities of Nazi Germany, that is, to man-made suffering, their thoughts remain pertinent to a world where most of humanity's suffering is brought about by human beings.

A crucial blow to the dual concept of the human body was delivered by the development of a phenomenology of the body initiated by Maurice Merleau-Ponty (1908-1961) in the wake of Husserl, and elaborated by scholars interested in the conjunction of the philosophy and ethics of medicine, presenting their thoughts in publications like the *Philosophy and*

## Medical Anthropology for Bioethics

*Medicine* series, *Medicine, Health Care and Philosophy, Journal of Medicine and Philosophy, Theoretical Medicine and Bioethics*, and contributions to leading relevant journals –*Bioethics, Developing World Bioethics, Journal of Medical Ethics*, among many others.

Flatly rejecting Cartesian dualism, phenomenologists understand the human body as a unity of the living and the lived body. The lived body

> Is bound up with, and directed toward, an experienced world. It is a being in relationship to that which is other: other people, other things, an environment. Moreover, in a significant sense, the lived body helps to constitute this world-as-experienced. We cannot understand the meaning and form of objects without reference to the bodily powers through which we engage them –our senses, motility, language, desires. The lived body is not just one thing *in* the world, but a way in which the world comes to be. (Leder 1992, 25)

The lived body perceives the world and elaborates the intentional project of acting in it by means of the living body that performs according to its corporeal possibilities and limitations. The living body is the organism, socially visible, medically observed and intervened. The process of lived experiences and corporeal practices is known as embodiment, "the lived fact of experiencing the world from and in and with just this body, my body" (Casey 2001, 206).

> Unwelcome as it has been, embodiment acts as a covert basis of human experience and a coherent connection among human beings: a basis and connection that occur not only in time but in space (and more particularly in place). (Ibid., 2007)

The world is perceived and embodied by the lived body, which corporeally transcends into the world by acts of exbodiment of the living body. For some reason, thoughts on embodiment have not considered the inverse corporeal act of "exbodiment", that is, the body itself –the body proper– creating culture. For example, there is quite convincing evidence that body laterality is overwhelmingly expressed as right-handedness;

actual right-sidedness is pre-cultural, appearing in various forms in a number of animal species. Humans have developed a culture of right-handedness (scissors, door handles, and many more man-made objects that vex the left-handed), even developing a value-laden description of the right-handed as dexterous (*dexter* = right), the lefties are sinister (Lat. *Sinister* = left).

The human body is becoming a favorite subject of philosophy (Marzano), sociology and anthropology (Le Breton), knitting a complex meshwork of reflection that, unfortunately, moves away from the pristine experience everyone has of the own body. In the religious sense, humans do not simply reproduce, they procreate; every zygote has the full ontological and moral status of a human being endowed with what Michael Sandel calls "the gifted quality of life". Secularity prefers to believe that embryos and fetuses acquire human status as they develop, just as human beings may be declared brain-dead even if certain basic functions of the living body are maintained beyond the irreversible loss of lived body activity.

Genetics and medicine have learned to repair the body, incorporate spare parts, transplant a fresh organ in exchange for the malfunctioning flesh of the diseased, and enhance the functionality of the body beyond the norm. All these matters that bioethics grapple with are doomed to unrelenting disagreement because the diverse initial premises of the body's significance are incompatible. Debates about the elusive nature of the human become more virulent as genetics and neuroscience are willing and able to reify human nature, as Habermas laments. If the idea of human nature flounders, the intrinsic value of dignity and human rights loses purchase and needs to be rethought.

Birth rites are performed as religious, familial and social recruitments, receiving the newborn –a cultural *tabula rasa*– as a member of a specific worldview impregnated with beliefs and meaning. In times of individualism and autonomy, precocious pre-voluntary initiations are rebelled against, shedding doctrines and militating against moral and social discriminations based on corporeal features. Independent of skin color, gender, ethnic features or functional limitations, the universal commonality

# Medical Anthropology for Bioethics

103

of the human body is requiring long overdue equal moral and social status and yet, the necessary reduction of power differentials is not happening. The quest for equality continues to be an unrealistic illusion, while an unrelenting imbalance of power renders the poor voiceless and neglected.

At best, it could be hoped that all humans *should* be treated as equals because they share certain fundamental anthropological attributes that are indispensable for survival and to face the vulnerabilities of the living body. Being born into the world with these transcendental anthropological features precedes the cultural development of the newborn, and they endure throughout a life that, if lived in good faith, will create its own meaning or voluntarily accept a significant offering doctrine, always resistant to a heteronomous indoctrination.

The quest for a pristine, pre-significant condition of the human body, begins by acknowledging that the one and only feature that all human bodies share is a human body with an equal universal ontological and moral status, precociously co-opted into contextual inequities and cultural appropriation operating even before birth. As things stand, if bioethics is to debate life and death issues concerning all human beings, as well as the ontological and moral status of the unborn, the life-threatening malformed, and the dying, it will have to search for the anthropological common traits that all humans share, which ought to remain undaunted throughout all stages and circumstances of each individual life.

Avoiding the dichotomous interplay between nature and culture, between individual psychophysical predispositions and the enormous constructive influence of society –Schütz, Berger and Luckmann–, embodiment explains the interaction between each human life and the world's anthropological quests, whether asking what or exploring who "man is", referring to the human body already situated in the world, embedded in processes of embodiment of culture and actively participating in society. To explore coming to be-in-the-world before being-in-the-world, is crucial to understand the formation of identity, and to acknowledge that the significance of human life is not a given; existence is a journey towards adopting or developing a meaning. Human beings that are rigidly co-opted into a worldview, be it secular or religious, what Max

Scheler called "the human place in the cosmos", are robbed of their existential choice to develop their own, singular existential intentionality, by placing their goals and answering to their particular set of values. All too often, circumstances and influences stunt the exploration of one's way and meanings.

> Because what they are in themselves is at any point the outcome of such a developmental process depending on their attitudes, essentially self-conscious beings do not have *natures*, they have *histories*. Or, put differently, it is their nature to have not just a *past*, but a *history*: a sequence of partially self-constituting self-transformations, mediated at every stage by their self-conceptions, and culminating in their being what they currently are. (Brandom 2011, 41)

## III. THE TRANSCENDENTAL ANTHROPOLOGICAL CONDITIONS OF THE HUMAN

Far from being an abstract entity, the human body is the concrete living realty of humans always situated in the world. To be born is to be placed in the world, what Heidegger briefly referred to as *Sein zum Anfang* –being-towards-beginning– on the way to his more crucial idea of *Sein zum Tode* –being-towards-death. Hannah Arendt highlights birth rather than death, based on "St. Augustine's indication that the divine creation of Man was for the human capacity to begin." The "fact of natality" gives birth to diverse individuals, to singular men, not to Man; before placing life's beginning in-the-world, natality inaugurates a free life. If singular human beings were born in freedom then truly every newborn would present in the world with equal rights and dignity (Vetter 2008, 138). As it stands, the idea is Arendt's post-Holocaust and anti-totalitarian wishful thinking.

The anthropological reality is that human beings are born into a world frozen in a *status quo*, as vulnerable beings dependent on others to survive in their given, not chosen, environment. They grow and mature to integrate

# Medical Anthropology for Bioethics

with their social milieu in order to develop their existence, a primary feat that requires certain transcendental –conditions of necessity– features that are universally present in every single human being: relationality, mundane transcendence, and transcendence of the self.

Every living body requires food, as well as shelter from destructive natural forces and predatory attacks, developing certain capabilities to survive. The human species has excelled at knowing and controlling nature by culture, which means that basic essential wants are no longer obtained by direct access to natural sources, but are almost exclusively mediated by social processes. It follows that anthropological wants are essential to satisfy biological needs and social integration. These essential anthropological features are present in each member of the species; human beings cannot survive in isolation and yet, living in society requires developing the transcendental attributes into competencies: relationality for cooperation, being-in-the-world to act in it, and transcendence of the self to grace life with continuity.

The human body is the basic commonality shared by all living members of our species, which survive and exist by externalizing towards others –relationality– and into the world where the living body labors, works and acts in pursuance of the identity and life-project of the lived body's existence. Every singular individual creates a self-conscious identity that posits itself, and is posited, in the world.

## A. Relationality

Relationality is at the core of personal identity, based as it is on recognition of the self and the other. The ideas of *homo sociologicus,* of social action as a fundamental inter-human activity, of speech as essential to cultural communication, and of dialogical ethics as the basis for morally relating to the other, all point in the same direction: humans relate to other humans. Relating is vitally essential, but it also is the source of unequal and damaging power relationships. Society bonds, but it also creates bondages and other spurious relations, like Hegel's master-slave relations,

# 106 *Miguel Kottow*

leonine contracts, and medical paternalism. In these asymmetric relations power often forces non-negotiable "take it or leave it" clauses to the detriment of the weaker parties, and it is the unavoidable tragedy of any social order that it functions on the basis of power differences that may be overturned, but never disappear.

Relationality has gained some academic attention in social studies where the term "relational turn" is suggested in order to stress the inter-human relations in social organization and institutions. Relationality has also become a prominent topic in feminist ethics –Gilligan, Noddings–, arguing that the masculine moral language –Kohlberg– pivots around justice and rule-compliance, whereas the feminine voice is more attuned to interpersonal relationships of compassion and care.

In the present context, relationality is to be understood as a pre-moral, and pre-social basic feature of human beings, a fact of natality that needs to be recognized, respected, and sustained in vulnerable life stages: immaturity, marginalization, and aging. "We need relationships, and we need relationships in which we count for something, relationships to which we can refer in order to define ourselves" (Bauman 2005, 68). Significant relationships require identity of those who relate, and identity is based on recognition and inclusion.

Interestingly, Martin Buber lecturing on "what is man" came to the conclusion that humanity is to be identified rather than described, and that man is the being who relates to the other –dialogical ethics–.

> Social connectedness has structural and functional dimensions. The structural dimension covers the quantity and form of a person's relationships, whereas the functional dimension covers the quality of those relationships and the support derived. (Stafford et al. 2018, 1)

Beyond its anthropological dimension, relationality means being acknowledged as social connectedness and its beneficial influence on prevention and the early detection of diseases.

Like most terms and ideas employed in non-empirical disciplines, relationality is deprived of meaning when presented as an isolated

## Medical Anthropology for Bioethics

107

foundational concept. Relational liberty, for example, is *"freedom through transactions and relationships of interdependency with others…*relational liberty is a practice of freedom that constitutes –and *is constituted by– membership,* by which I mean participatory parity and equality of civic respect" (Jennings 2015, 10). Relationality is certainly pregnant with meanings that go beyond the transcendental anthropological feature of the human being as here presented.

## B. Mundane Transcendence

In its most usual and forthright connotation, transcendence refers to a realm beyond the material world, of a metaphysical nature and habitually related to a divine force. In the current age of secular culture, transcendence is often employed to describe the individual stepping into the world, what Martha Nussbaum depicts as transcendence of an *internal kind;* in this view, more ethical than anthropological, internal or mundane transcendence is a passage from ordinary life to the display of excellence. But transcendence is not a virtue, it is an unavoidable and vitally indispensable positioning of the human existence entering the world and becoming part of it. Mundane transcendence can, but need not, expand into the belief of an eternal form of transcendence. Not explored here is an interesting line of thought based on the Marxian idea of alienation and reification that capitalism imposes on human beings existing in a technified world that maims relationality by reducing interaction with significant others, and narrows mundane transcendence by eroding the difference between objects and subjects that turn into a composite of facts and fetishes that Bruno Latour calls "factishes."

> Reification affects relations between persons, and even within the person: one becomes an object to oneself, self-alienated as well as alienated from other humans, particularly those with whom we should be expressing class solidarity.

108          *Miguel Kottow*

> This implies that objects are transformed into subjects and subjects are turned into objects, with the result that subjects are rendered passive or determined, while objects are rendered as the active, determining factors. (Jeffreys 2016, 86)

Philosophy is purportedly a clarifying enterprise but in fact it shows a tiresome tendency towards unveiling or creating complexities. Thinking about the limits of the body, the idea of the "body-subject of the world" crops up to confuse a limit between the body and the world "lost in the folds of a common element from which both devolve, making it difficult to see where one ends and the other begins or draw any clear distinction between that which belongs to the body and that which belongs to the world" (Abrahamsson and Simpson 2011, 334). Nothing could be further from the experience of identity, individuality, and self, showing how disquisitions may wander from reality and become unenlightening.

## C. Transcendence of the Self

As the identity of the self develops the individual immersed in social relations and self-conscious agency of being-in-the-world develops a sense of direction. Every act is an anticipation of the present into the future, employing the means to reach a desired goal. The concatenation of acts inspired in a sense of values unfolds into a meaningful life. Ideally, human life should not have an externally imposed meaning, for it is a prerogative of every singular individual to search for significance in his own life. Whatever each person strives to accomplish, it will be accompanied by the hope of persistence, a sense of achievement that survives after death, the quest to leave a mark, a legacy, a post-mortal presence: having children, creating a work of art, participating in social, political, or religious movements, being remembered in the family photo album:

> In the modern solution, immortality is transferred from the realm of preordained fate to that of achievement: and a kind of achievement that in principle would be never final and definite.

*Medical Anthropology for Bioethics* 109

> One can hedge one's bet, trying to behave in what the opinions of the times consider the best way to earn a place in the grateful memory of posterity, but no more than that. (Bauman and Raud 2005, 10)

Biotechnology is offering opportunities to outwit mortality by cryopreservation, stem-cell banking, longevity and other technical tricks, thus unwillingly making the point that the body might eventually outlive its death, but failing to imagine possible distortions of self-identity in an artificially preserved or renewed living body.

As Western culture developed the idea of self-contained individuality unfettered by otherworldly transcendence, modern existence sought to ignore the final void of death. If *Dasein* is being-towards-death, perhaps this can be interpreted as striving to take the edge off death's total annihilation of *Dasein*. The wish to transcend the self beyond biological finitude has many faces, fitting easily into traditions that see each life as enmeshed with nature and concatenated in an uninterrupted participation with one's ancestors. Oriental and many ethnic cultures do not worry about transcendence of the self, for they are connected with the world beyond death. For them, individuality is selfish.

Every human is born with the anthropological features that, unless thwarted or not developed, are indispensable to survive among one's fellow men. Given that birth is radically contextual, every human being will relate and transcend under different circumstances. Natality is always involved in disparity, in inequity that will breed further injustice, so the idea that all human beings are equal is irresponsibly vacuous. The British anthropologist Marylin Strathern is quoted as stating: "It is the middle class that makes a project out of life." Those that have not reached this social condition remain entrapped in a permanent struggle to survive, and have little strength or means to engage in project-searching, while those belonging to the privileged class enjoy financial independence and freedom of choice that allow them to satisfy their desires without having to make long-term goal commitments.

But transcend we all must, by relating and coming to be in the midst of our contextualized social reality where biological needs are to be satisfied.

In other words, anthropology is always situational (Figure 1). Those deprived of the anthropologically mediated basic biological needs, fall from the state of *bios* into that of *zoe*, losing their humanity and being reduced to mere animality, a horrifying reality staged in concentration camps, prisons, and absolute poverty. Most unfortunately, similar degradations occur in our midst, as has been reported about old-fashioned psychiatric institutions and hospices.

Inversely, those acquiring well-being and wealth may well reduce and select their relationality, becoming impervious and insensitive, condemning any unwanted contacts to be unheard and neglected. The rich tend to channel and isolate their mundane transcendence to the point of seclusion and eccentricity –the cloistered elite, the ghettos of the rich–. The marginal poor and the isolated rich have a fractured relationality and mundane transcendence, failing to engage in the basic ethical concerns required to survive in a decent –self-satisfying– manner.

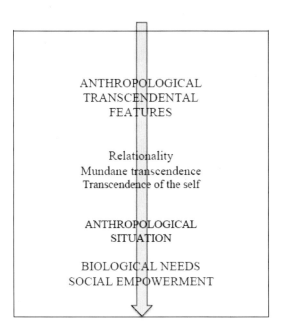

Figure 1. Schematic representation of transcendental anthropological features mediating biological needs and social empowerment through relationality and mundane transcendence.

# IV. ANTHROPOLOGY AS HEURISTICS OF FEAR

In his famous book *The Imperative of Responsibility*, Hans Jonas (1903-1993) laments the absence of an ethics for the distant and theoretical isolation of moral responsibility. Before attending our wishes for a future, of which we know so little, the heuristic of fear ought to be cultivated so as to avoid the worst, the extinction of humankind by the uncontrolled excesses of biotechnoscience. Knowing thy threats and risks is a variation of Jonas' heuristic of fear, yet it points in the same direction, that human nature, although undetermined, ought to be preserved.

Stimulating fear may well be a double-edged sword by combining stressful concern for a negative future with the Cassandra syndrome voiced by environmentalists alerting us to impending catastrophes, which, true or exaggerated, are profusely exposed but rarely headed in a substantial way. Fear mongering is also at the base of talk about sustainable growth, usually countered by faith in technology to neutralize the damage it creates.

In his pioneering book *Bioethics. Bridge to the Future*, Van Renselaer Potter wrote: "The purpose of this book is to contribute to the future of the human species by promoting the formation of a new discipline, the discipline of *Bioethics*." He also included a Bioethical Creed for Individuals, the second of which states:

> Belief: I accept the fact that the future survival and development of mankind, both culturally and biologically, is strongly conditioned by man's present activities and plans.
>
> Commitment: I will try to live my own life and to influence the lives of others so as to promote the evolution of a better world for future generalizations of mankind, and I will try to avoid actions that would jeopardize their future. (Potter 1971)

Potter was profoundly influenced by deep ecologist Aldo Leopold, in his demand to respect nature and to instrumentalize whatever needs to be done in order to develop a "new wisdom that will provide the 'knowledge of how to use knowledge' for man's survival and for improvement in the quality of life" (Ibid., 1). Videotaping a presentation at the 4th World Congress on Bioethics, Potter proclaimed: "Global Bioethics, as a new Science Ethics, is required for long-term Human Survival." Unquestionably an anthropocentric ethics, Potter's global ethics was adopted by eco-ethicists who posited that biodiversity and the harmonious conservation of nature had intrinsic value not to be ignored by human interests.

In a blog on biodiversity, a picture of flowering cacti is shown with the caption: "The cactus is one of the species with intrinsic value as it has no value for humans." Beneath it, another image depicts a leopard carrying its dead prey, footed by the caption "Hunting by the wild animals is an unethical intrinsic value required for the balance in biodiversity" (Biodiversity 2010). "Unethical intrinsic value" is a contradiction in terms.

What remains stable beyond the debate of defense and respect for the intrinsic value of biodiversity versus the fundamental value of humanity is survival. Human action and knowledge must avoid imprudently exploiting nature, but the point of global ethics is finally, in Potter's concept, not biodiversity *per se* but "long-term human survival." Digging deeper into these controversies shows a profound cut severing the belief in the exceptionality of the human that must be preserved at all cost since it represents the summit of biological development, from those who see no reason to hinder the development of a superhuman or post-human being.

In an as yet unpublished article, the Danish scholar Peter Kemp describes three major realms of ethical thought: interpersonal, anthropological and, with the advent of biotechnical and especially genetic developments, a post-anthropological current of ethics that irradiates towards life and nature, that he calls "anthropocentrifugal", meaning that ethics cannot but be posited by human beings. A more proper term might be anthropogenic, which is equally applicable to Aristotelian virtue ethics or the theological or postmodern ethic, since any kind of ethics will be man-made.

Consequently, the idea that contemporaneous Western ethics has evolved from a body-centered anthropological fundament to a biotechnologically induced "anthropocentrifugal" perspective, means that

*Medical Anthropology for Bioethics* 113

bioethics addresses human intervention in life and nature, all endowed with an intrinsic value that makes them indestructible. Ethics is unavoidably a human construct, therefore always anthropogenic, which does not mean that it needs to be anthropocentric although, in the ultimate analysis, its core is always the survival of humanity. The unacknowledged debt of environmental, global, or any other holistic form of ethics is to first salvage actual suffering humanity before pouring eulogies onto biodiversity, sustainability, justice, the gift of life, and so on, all praiseworthy and highly valuable, provided the man-made unhappiness of the many is attended to.

*Chapter 6*

# ETHICS AND NEGLECTED DISEASES

## I. ETHICAL ASPECTS

Ethics purports to evaluate human action by making a distinction between right and wrong, based on a variety of values and priorities nested in different worldviews and basic notions about human nature. As societies become more complex, beliefs and certitudes multiply leading to diverse and often conflictive views of right and wrong. Max Weber (1864-1920) concluded that traditional ethics of conviction had to be enriched, perhaps even replaced, by an ethics of responsibility, for acting upon beliefs affects others and has to be accounted for. Currently, ethics is understood as reflecting on human actions performed in liberty –freely chosen– and with responsibility –accountable to others–.

Philosophers from Aristotle to Mill have developed intricate systems of ethics condensed under three headings: Virtue ethics –aretology–, deontology or duty-based ethics, and utilitarianism or consequentialism, that consider the best action as the one that maximizes utility for the most. In the actual world we inhabit, says A. MacIntyre, the language of morality is in "grave disorder", not surprisingly when recounting the horrors of two world wars, the development of atomic destruction, ecological man-made disasters, technoscientific expansion manipulating nature and human biology, and the fathomless divide between the few haves and the majority of deprived and underprivileged human beings.

Recent decades have witnessed the emergence of a non-affirmative brand of ethics based on the idea that life is a vale of suffering, where the least and only duty of everyone is to avoid harming others. Without overtly saying so, negative ethics rejects any commitment to the common weal and remains indifferent to suffering. Negativity is the breeding ground of neglect, unaware that ignoring bad lives is in itself harmful. Furthermore, negative ethics cannot dismiss Apel's thought that talking about ethics, even in a disparaging way, is already an ethical act of communication and debate –pragmatic transcendentalism–. As far as human beings are necessarily embedded in society, they can only integrate, interact and survive by accepting a "fundamental ethical articulation", as Argentinian philosopher Julio Cabrera calls the basic duty of not harming others. The social exchange of communication, goods and services can only occur if a basis of honest decency is presupposed and practiced.

The collapse of normative ethics and some of its most cherished tools –universal principles, consensus seeking practices, participatory decision-making, the sacredness of human nature, a limitless respect for biodiversity–, opened the need to address particular moral issues in private and public life, giving birth to applied ethics concerned with actual quandaries that require morally defensible decisions. Lacking ethical principles, dominant ideas of tolerance, pluralism and autonomy were hailed, challenging democratic societies to secure a multicultural common public morality. Substantive debates gave way to procedural claims for universal participation, communicative discourse ethics (Habermas, Apel), the exercise of reflective equilibrium in the quest for a fair society (Rawls), or coherentism as the balance between top-down and bottom-up models of discourse (T. Beauchamp). Procedural proposals remain enclosed in airtight compartments theorizing about rational deliberating monads that ignore the reality of living bodies existing within specific social and cultural contexts: "Habermas fails to grasp adequately the significance of the embodied, situational and dialogical elements of everyday human life", as M. Gardiner writes in praise of Mikhail Bakhtin's "phenomenology of 'practical doing', one that focuses on our incarnated activities within the lifeworld" (Gardiner 2004, 32).

*Ethics and Neglected Diseases*

Reaching out for universality cultivates an abstractness that is irrelevant to the concrete contexts of actual life, and the individuality of full-blooded human bodies intent on living their existential identity.

> If we do not allow moral values or self-interest to corrupt the delivery of the just and legal delivery of health services, we should not let other values, such as religious values, corrupt them either. (Savulescu 2006, 295)

## II. SOLIDARITY

Solidarity is called upon whenever the ethical aspects of a collective or global issue are under debate. The nature of solidarity is hard to pin down: Is it a virtue, an instrument to assist other virtues, social capital, an inherent feature of collective life, or is it a vacuous idea that is nice to talk about yet impossible to realize? Does a variation of Thomas's sociological theorem apply? If people define solidarity as real, is it real in its consequences? Definitions are of little help: "concerned with human well-being", "merely one way of organizing our social institutions", "a certain kind of cooperation", and "acts carried out to support others", are a sample culled by Prainsack and Buyx 2011, 2016), giving the impression that solidarity is an idea that is unable to stand by itself, rather acting as a decorative element in other concepts concerned with public relationships. The tacit and ancillary character of solidarity shows how undetermined the concept is: "We define solidarity as a moral practice that is fundamental to a social and cultural structure of right relationship" (Jennings and Dawson 2015, 32).

More to the present point is to briefly explore whether solidarity is in any of its understandings a descriptive or prescriptive way of attaching it to the problem of neglected populations, a query that depends on the perspective adopted. Solidarity is often seen as a "moral/ethical value" captured by its emphasis on "community, equality and the active promotion of welfare" and "may require collective interests to take priority

118                      *Miguel Kottow*

over the interests of individuals or sub-collectives" (Harmon 2006, 216, 217)

> Solidarity is a moral vehicle for injecting legitimate concepts and considerations of community and interconnectedness into ethical and legal analyses. If the potential benefits of solidarity are to be realized (e.g., redressing some of the shortcomings of the existing healthcare deficit), solidarity must be ranked with other popularly claimed and largely complimentary moral values such as sanctity of life and human dignity. (Ibid., 221)

Solidarity means connectedness in pursuit of a common goal by active support, deploying a form of "strong solidarity" that specifies how and for whom the potential benefits of solidary actions are meant. In contrast, "weak solidarity consists in *the willingness to take the perspective of others seriously*" (Gunson 2009, 247). Taking the perspective of others has a long history in psychology, child development and the social construction of reality, strongly emphasizing the cognitive aspects of relating to others. Solidarity is recognized as a European sociopolitical issue that inspired the realization of postwar welfare nations, but its survival as a social force, if it ever was one, is much endangered by contemporary individualism, the feebleness of the State, and a growing trend towards aggressive competitiveness and irrational consumer binges.

Tax schemes or collective insurance schemes claiming solidarity are truly financial impositions needed to balance duties of delivery for those who are entitled but unable to pay, by raising capital at the expense of wealthier people. This crude devaluation of solidarity comes to mind when reading about "the role of the state in helping to institutionalise and to enforce solidaristic arrangements" (Prainsac and Buyx 2011, 29). The idea of enforcing solidarity is an oxymoron illustrating the inflationary use of an elusive concept. Commenting on the "problematic character of the solidarity concept" these authors suggest that "Perhaps it is indeed the case that a 'solidarity inversion exists' –the more solidaristic we are, the less we talk about it" (Ibid., 38). Just as plausibly, the inversion can be inverted: the more we talk about solidarity, the less we practice it, at least in times of

*Ethics and Neglected Diseases*									119

peace and quiet. Crises like war, and natural catastrophes will stimulate short-lived acts of solidarity, which are hard to find in modern individualism.

Solidarity has not figured prominently in bioethics. Calling for "greater imaginative creativity", a four-tiered concept of solidarity is suggested:

> We propose to explore solidarity as a concept having four dimensions: one foundation and three relational dimensions. The foundational dimension is solidarity as a form of *standing up beside.* The three relational dimensions are *standing up for, standing up with,* and *standing up as.* (Jennings and Dowson 2015, 35)

Paraphrasing Martha Nussbaum's treatment of dignity, solidarity perhaps should not be seen as a foundational concept, but rather as forming part of a network of related notions (Jennings 2015).

## III. ETHICAL BLINDNESS

Ethical blindness is the inability to see the ethical dimension of a decision at stake, even failing to perceive the ethical dimension of real situations. Invisibility may occur when euphemistic language has caused ethical issues to fade away, or may be induced by rigid framing, i.e., seeing problems from one perspective without being aware that other viewpoints also exist. For example, if big business justifies its huge profit by claiming to be under a moral obligation to its shareholders, it will fail to acknowledge the existence of other duties that should deserve moral consideration, like the endangered accessibility to high-priced essential goods. As previously presented, neglected diseases are prone to invisibility, except for macrostatistics that rely on incomplete data given that nations harboring poverty and neglect are in no position to comprehensively survey their territory in order to obtain complete and reliable data collections. In fact, large-number statistics tend to hide differences and make extremes invisible: A Gini index does not inform about precarious subsistence income or the lack of it, nor does the count of over 800 million people suffering from hunger give a vivid picture of a child dying of starvation. The problematic reality of neglected diseases needs to be recognized in its true demographic dimensions as well as in the depth of individual suffering.

Ethical blindness prevails as long as other points of view are too weak to kindle and activate the moral imagination about unheeded values that ought to be considered, helping to replace rigid framings with flexible ones. "The most effective cure for ethical blindness is an atmosphere of open, democratic, and critical deliberation" (Palazzo, Krings and Hoffrage 2013, 14).

A subtle but telling difference exists between invisibility and neglect. Ethical blindness is amenable to education and persuasion, it is a defective perception without moral implications, as compared to ethically responsible neglect causing harm that can and should be mitigated.

Ethical blindness is mainly discussed in business ethics and, inasmuch as the pharmaceutical industry is a paradigm of big business, these considerations apply and are sharpened by the question of the moral duty of healthcare providers.

## IV. NEGLECTED DISEASES: LIFTING THE VEIL

In a very coarse outline, the realities of neglected diseases can be seen as problems of disparity in the availability of medical and preventive healthcare, and intentional indifference to the research and development of effective agents to mitigate or eliminate hitherto unattended diseases.

The concept of neglected diseases includes a number of very distinct conditions, often lumped together in a way that ignores the diversity of approaches required to evaluate them and bring to light their specific needs, as becomes apparent in the variety of descriptions presented.

Neglected diseases are "those that primarily affect populations with little purchasing power, and therefore offer an insufficient incentive for industry to invest in R&D" (Moon, Bermudez and t'Hoen 2012). In a blog entry, the psychiatrist and public health specialist Dr. Layla McCay states: "In terms of the science, it seems that 'rare diseases' are more likely to be neglected than so-called 'neglected tropical diseases.'"

Neglected diseases have become naturalized as an inevitable consequence of adverse socioeconomic determinants that cause and maintain appalling levels of poverty, condemning vast populations to dire life conditions lacking preventive public health measures, access to effective medication, and a sharply curtailed life expectancy as compared to developed countries. Public health specialist T. McKeown famously showed that the prevalence of infectious diseases tended to decline as living standards improved, long before specific vaccines and antibiotic therapies were developed. The inverse situation is not symmetrical: poverty continues to breed endemic and epidemic infections, but vaccines and antibiotics do exist, though are not available to the destitute, thus explaining the persistence of neglected diseases.

> Neglected tropical diseases (NTDs) is an umbrella term for a diverse group of debilitating infections that represent the most common afflictions for 2.7 billion people living on less than U.S. $2 per day. (Bernhard, Houghton and Teplitskaya 2014, 162)

Healthcare disparities range from boutique medicine, enhancement interventions, medicalization and overmedication, to the total lack of biomedical care. The resurgence of alternative medicines and of healing practices rooted in ethnic traditions is a partial and insufficient substitute for absent allopathic medicine. Therapeutic drugs are allopathic medicine's strongest assets predominantly provided by pharmaceutical enterprises, and it is anticipated that their price will increase substantially in coming years, as R&D becomes more sophisticated, therefore more costly, and less efficient. The search for new antibiotics, for example, has not been very successful, whereas some of the biggest blockbusters are the product of serendipitous findings (sildenafil (Viagra), Methylphenidate (Ritalin)). Even well-funded public health vaccination programs need to deal with local realities where cosmologies may be reticent to comply, or distances and travelling costs conspire to the misuse of antibiotics and incomplete immunization, thus contributing to the re-emergence of diseases and resistant strains of pathogens (Das 1999).

Dragging R&D initiatives to prevent, mitigate or eventually cure neglected and rare diseases maximizes profits at the cost of prolonged suffering, creating a major problem for ethics given that large private enterprises continue to devise and step up mostly those strategies that secure huge profits at all costs. Profit-motivated tactics in postponing innovation where it is most needed remain impervious to ethical approaches urging the lessening of injustice in healthcare for the underprivileged.

## V. Awareness of Harm

Economic proposals to reinvent the presence of the neglected diseases based on incentives, private-public associations and governmental initiatives to share benefits between profiteers and the needy, have had a positive effect in some important instances, but remain insufficient to mollify widespread and entrenched healthcare neglect.

Apart from some sporadic and rapidly dwindling sparks of interest in the problems of severe health and healthcare problems affecting the poor, the issue of neglected diseases was not raised to extended concern till the beginning of the present century, as the world realized that "Neglected tropical diseases represent the most common diseases for the 2·7 billion people living on less than US$2 per day." The initial studies emphasizing healthcare neglect specifically identify three levels of neglect that are common to all the targeted diseases—local, national, and international. In a later approach, definitions centered on diseases' shared sociomedical features and their effects on poverty and development have been discussed (Liese and Schubert 2009; Liese, Rosenberg and Schratz 2010).

A "multi-stakeholder" meeting closely connected to the WHO's 2020 Roadmap on NTDs came up with the "London Declaration on Neglected Tropical Diseases" (2010), committed to controlling and eradicating ten of the most devastating NTDs by 2020. Acknowledging the need to "provide the resources necessary across sectors to remove the primary risk factors for NTD –poverty and exposure–", the document relies heavily on supplying and extending "drug access programmes" and "advancing R&D" (www.who.int/neglected_diseases/London_Declaration_NTDs.pd).

Despite hailing the London Declaration as "monumental" in its commitments and goals, critical reflection concludes that "Though scientific progress in addressing some infectious diseases is moving forward, the goals of elimination and eradication of all NTDs remain largely distant", thus tempering but neither contradicting nor discouraging the admirable efforts to combat NTDs on many fronts, as well as recognizing that "some progress has been made towards treating, controlling, eliminating, and possibly eradicating certain NTDs" (Mackey et al. 2014). A number of scholars have confirmed that "substantial achievements" through increasing drug donations by pharmaceutical companies were reported, but Official Development Assistance (ODA), largely provided by the U.S. and the U.K., has notoriously stagnated (Liese, Houghton and Tepliskaya 2014).

The challenges of reducing the burdens of NTDs are multiple and require the cooperation of many stakeholders, developing a variety of strategies that need to be flexible and adaptable to different diseases and to many social, economic, geographic, and environmental realities.

> NTDs are addressed through five strategies: preventive chemotherapy, intensified disease management, vector control, veterinary public health measures for zoonotic neglected diseases, and through improved water and sanitation.
>
> Disease-specific alliances generate opportunities for advocacy and increased resources from non-traditional donors, and reflect the need to facilitate interaction between endemic countries, international organisations, non-governmental organisations, pharmaceutical donors, philanthropic foundations, and academia. (Molineux, Savioli, Engels 2017, 312)

Medical, public health and general healthcare issues would seem to be adequately tackled with performance and achievement policies, but need to be guided by ethical motivation to avoid perversions and distortions such as market-oriented practices, severely skewed benefit/costs evaluations, and a biased promotion of interests that are contrary to requirements of the common weal.

Programs directed at treating and preventing neglected diseases have sought a direct impact on the proximal causes of infection, contagion and epidemic spreading, which are important to reduce disease burdens, but lose purchase when socioeconomic causes of poverty and healthcare disparities remain unchanged or even worsened.

Pathologies of power, structural violence, globalization and its consequent increase of inequality, as well as dwindling public support for the underprivileged, are huge processes that respond to factors that a critical theory is incapable of fully grasping though, to be in any way coherent, a *status quo* that serves the interests of a mere segment of humanity must time and again be intellectually challenged and disparaged.

Major interventions require the teaming up of tremendous financial and technical resources engaged in a common cause of resolving the most severe healthcare problems of modern times. Nevertheless, should instrumental reason continue to prevail without being inspired by respect and concern for humanity's common weal, current pragmatic powers would keep on benefiting the actual dominant technoscientific approach to the detriment of the less fortunate.

*Chapter 7*

# COPING WITH NEGLECTED POPULATIONS

## I. BRINGING NEGLECT ISSUES TO THE FORE

Generalized discomfort and concern about worldwide growing inequality and social injustice have been chronically lip-serviced, with a tendency to naturalize absolute poverty and unmet basic needs in populated underdeveloped regions subject to equally naturalized socioeconomic determinants. Recent awareness is rekindled by the encroachment of dire living conditions in well-off societies threatened by the unstable and decreasing well-being of the middle-classes caught in the throng of relative poverty –stagnating salaries, insolvency and the privatization of public social services–, together with growing healthcare neglect in the midst of wealthy nations turning into blue marble health regions. Concern at the menace of the worldwide spread of epidemics –HIV, SARS, $H_1N_1$, Ebola, perhaps dengue in the near future– is sporadically unsettling the hitherto protected.

Circumstantial and sketchy concerns explain the lack of coherent and sustained measures to redress injustice and temper globalization's impact on disparity and insecurity. In healthcare and the issues of neglected diseases, well-meant proposals and programs are unable to counter the forces of medicalization and the siphoning of resources towards overuse.

The insatiable profiteering of managed medicine and pharmaceutical empires, supported by successful lobbying has weakened corrective approaches –DOHA–, allowed deregulations –TRIPs plus– and legislated in favor of the powerful –patent laws, unfair FTAs, and the reduction of budgets for public health and national healthcare systems–.

Neglected diseases constitute a political, social and economic conundrum of problems converging to an essential ethical issue of rampant unfairness. The structural forces involved are neither abstract nor theoretical, they are potent conditioners strung along a chain of well-identified policies, especially for the pharmaceutical and medical instrumental supplies industries (Pogge 2008):

- Increasing corporate earnings by securing the monopoly of products.
- Disease mongering.
- International money loans requiring fiscal austerity and the market presence of healthcare.
- Siphoning resources from poor economies through the sale of armaments.
- Energy savings through biofuels that make food less available and more expensive.
- TRIPs and TRIPs plus agreements.
- R&D captured by such strategies as the 10/90 divide, the offshoring of research, and the employment of CROs.

At best, one-third of the world's population enjoys some financial security, social welfare and the benefits of technoscientific innovations. The worse-off one-third lives in dire need, insecure and unprotected, and suffering from at least one neglected disease, often up to five conditions that could be prevented or cured if innovation, availability and accessibility of preventive and therapeutics agents were targeted to their benefit. Lack of assistance and empowerment perpetuates socially induced pauperism and disease, conditions that cannot be hoped to improve spontaneously, letting events take their natural course, as Hippocrates managed diseases –

# Coping with Neglected Populations

the *vis medicatrix naturae–*. Hegel denied the healing power of nature, teaching that things will not adjust by themselves because order does not emerge spontaneously in society. But of course, the miseries of inequality are not natural; they are man-made afflictions and consequently constitute ethical misdeeds that no one is willing to account for. Although possible mitigations and solutions will depend on economic redistribution either in fairness or in the satisfaction of basic needs, the initial and sustained impulse can come from no other than an ethical source inspired to avoid maleficence and promote redress in recognition. Médecins Sans Frontières and many other nongovernmental organizations (NGOs) and the tireless commitment of individuals like Paul Farmer and Partners in Health, are admirably dedicated to providing healthcare for poor patients, but all these initiatives give relief without having the force, except by setting an example, to approach structural forces and demand profound changes in worldwide inequities and man-made vulnerabilities and harm.

There is no way of gauging how effective –problem solving– and efficient –cost/benefit relation– all these efforts and programs are, and it certainly is too soon to confirm sustained results when tackling such huge issues as NTDs. There is some heartening news on the eradication of lymphatic filariasis through mass drug administration in Togo, or the elimination of trachoma as a public health problem in Mexico, Morocco and Oman, moving the WHO to verbose expressions like "unprecedented, record-breaking progress." There also are some severe drawbacks, like the rapidly increasing spread of dengue, and the rising problem of emergent and re-emergent diseases. The changing nature of NTDs also merits further concern, as does the euphemistic approach to, and the whitewashing practice of, dubious and harmful policies as well as market-driven strategies in science, the transmission of knowledge and profit-oriented drug and medical devices companies. Recursively, technical solutions are expanded, opening new research horizons:

> Implementation research is important in global health because it addresses the challenges of the know-do gap in real-world settings and the practicalities of achieving national and global health goals... This

128 *Miguel Kottow*

Health Policy paper is part of a call to action to increase the use of implementation research in global health, build the field of implementation research inclusive of research utilisation efforts, and accelerate efforts to bridge the gap between research, policy, and practice to improve health outcomes. (Theobald et al. 2018)

## II. INITIAL APPROACHES

The time was ripe to generate new ways of approaching the implications, aspects, and consequences of leading-edge biomedical research explosively being developed by genetics. Bioethics was not up to the task, as shown by the Human Genome Project that declared it would devote 5% of its research budget to a newly conceived program called ELSI: Ethical, Legal and Social Implications of life sciences research, shortly to be followed by its European equivalent ELSA that prefers the more neutral term "aspects" over "implications". These programs took it upon themselves to increase public participation and interdisciplinary interaction –including the social sciences and the humanities– with the aim of expanding the diverse perspectives and amplifying the presence of actual and future stakeholders, though they persist in being welded to instrumental pragmatism.

Society should have a say in how the money is invested, i.e., transmutated into knowledge (which, hopefully, and eventually, can be transmutated back into money once again, through a process which is now often referred to as 'valorisation'). Moreover, society will function as the future *consumer* of the scientific knowledge thus produced, and as the *future* for new technological devices. (Zwart, Landeweerd and van Rooij 2014, 9)

Three basic approaches have been presented to face the problem of neglected and rare diseases, besides the as yet unfulfilled ethical and bioethical task of making them visible in all their magnitude and depth (see Chapter 8). Most vocally, global ethics, human rights and humanitarian

*Coping with Neglected Populations* 129

approaches have been summoned as elements to construct a globally just world. Secondly, many proposals respect the commercial thrust of healthcare providers, suggesting plans to reduce market prices and incentivize undiminished revenues by way of complex compensation programs to secure Big Pharma's revenues; the third approach decries big earnings in healthcare as unethical as long as they obstruct the availability of and access to medical and public health needs.

Holistic approaches:
- Global ethics and universal human rights
- Humanitarian assistance
- Solidarity and altruism

Incentive-based approaches
- R&D pull/push mechanisms
- Global Health Fund
- Advanced Market Commitment
- Health Impact Fund

Ethics-based approaches
- Moral duty to assist
- Moral assistance to the distant
- Bioethics

# III. GLOBAL ETHICS AND HUMAN RIGHTS

The WHO makes repeated efforts to relate human rights with neglected diseases, pointing at the growing attention to neglected tropical diseases as both a public health and a human rights issue. The right of health –the highest attainable standard of health– encompasses "underlying determinants of health", and "health care" interacting by means of four vectors: availability, accessibility, acceptability and quality. This theoretical framework "requires that health interventions support the capacity of duty bearers (primarily government authorities) to meet their obligations and of affected communities to claim their rights" (http://www.who.int/gender-equity-rights/knowledge/ntd-information-sheet-eng.pdf?ua=1).

The way to global bioethics is lit by the expectations of problem-solving scientific progress and the artificial enhancement of human attributes that promise a happy new world and an increased quality of life for those who can afford it. Francis Bacon's idea that science will benefit humanity is being distorted into serving the better off in a neoliberal globalization that increases inequalities at the cost of low-income populations.

For decades, progressive realization was understood as an aspirational commitment to advance economic, social and cultural (ESC) rights at the pace of national and economic development, while civil and political rights were to be implemented without delay. When it became clear that distinguishing two types of rights was increasing discrimination and inequality, the U.N. made a turnabout to reunite the drive to realize ESC and civil and political rights, but the damage was done and ESC rights continued to depend on national economic growth with the danger which is becoming real, that compliance to positive rights would regress in economic crises or slowed growth. The idea of progressive realization, *de jure* discredited, remained *de facto* in full vigor, oblivious to the ethical requirement that realization should not depend on economic statistics and data, but be sensitive to a legal framework supporting the human rights of the citizenry (Porter 2015).

Possibly aware of not having given more than cursory attention to the plight of neglected populations and neglected diseases, the WHO repeatedly summarizes and up-dates its sporadic concerns in the bland and uncommitted language it cannot dispense with.

The right to health is freely proclaimed in a variety of ways, ranging from "the right to a decent minimum of health care", to the right to the highest attainable standard of health extended to the "underlying determinants of health (i.e., access to education, clean water, housing, etc.)." Based on a never clearly defined "right to health", official WHO documents state that

*Coping with Neglected Populations* 131

The right to health care calls for immediate and targeted steps to be taken to progressively ensure that health services, goods and facilities are *available, accessible, acceptable and of good quality.*

A human rights-based approach requires that the interventions and processes in response to neglected tropical diseases are guided by human rights principles, such as *participation, non-discrimination and accountability.* (WHO 2009)

These somewhat tautological statements are topped by another truism: "Neglected diseases are both a cause and consequence of human rights violations." Chartering human rights and blaming all kinds of woes on non-compliance and violations of these rights have little instrumental value beyond their politically correct and largely uncontested approval. This may have been a motive for the "Universal Declaration on Bioethics and Human Rights" (see Chapter 1-II), and a stimulus to prioritize ethical reflections on the issue of neglect and healthcare.

The call for "reasonableness" in accelerating the pace towards fortifying institutions devoted to healthcare, social security, and cultural subsidies without compromising economic development through radical restructuring of national economies, increasing state resources by higher taxations and the reduction of military expenses, is very unlikely to happen. Rather, the cleft between good intentions and required policy changes contrary to neoliberalism and globalization is widening, gnawing at the credibility of thoughtful discourse faced with unrelenting political action. To the minds of many, political programs are being replaced by noisy populisms promising more than they can handle.

## IV. HUMANITARIAN APPROACHES

The immense majority of debates and policies directed at the need to free a third of the world population from its dire conditions of healthcare neglect have been based on economic schemes that might increase the medical assistance to the poor living in neglected populations or amidst the

132 *Miguel Kottow*

wealthy blue marble nations. Except for some notable successes to control specific infectious diseases in some low-income countries, overall results are unremarkable and slow, forcing the conclusion that the global problems of neglected diseases continue to be massive and largely unresponsive to tactics that assist without empowering, partially mitigating some aspects but also exacerbating others like the spread of resistant vectors and causal agents, increased contagiousness due to travel, migrations and urbanization, negatively contributing to the mounting problem of re-emergent, drug-resistant diseases.

Cloaked as humanitarian actions and systems, international aid has been criticized for imposing foreign values and renewing neo-colonial practices. "In the humanitarian programme cycle, there is no space for the long term –it is fast-paced, top-down and resource-heavy" (Jayawickrama 2018). Humanitarian aid is being studied by French sociologists and anthropologists, developing a "political anthropology of international aid [that] must take into account the current context of neo-liberal globalization –and subject it to rigorous and critical political analysis" (Atlani-Duault and Dozon 2011, VII). The French anthropologist Didier Fassin, at times closely linked to Médecins Sans Frontières, has thoroughly analyzed humanitarian intervention in war, though stating that it also has

> Become an important and even a dominant frame of reference for Western political intervention in global scenes of misfortune both in cases of armed conflict and natural disasters and around their more or less direct consequences in the form of epidemics, famine, physical injury and emotional trauma. (Fassin 2007, 508)

There is a "triple problematic of the humanitarian politics of life": the distinction between lives that may be risked from lives that can only be sacrificed, the separation of lives with higher value –international agents– and those receiving limited protection –local staff– and, third, the testimonial value even when circumstances hinder their active aid. "Humanitarian action by non-governmental organizations" distinguishes itself from those who "promote indifference to distant others" (Ibid., 518).

"Testimony has traditionally had a privileged relationship to the body and within the medicalised tint of humanitarianism the suffering body has always had particular salience" (Reid-Henry 2013, 759). The rejection of indifference –neglect–, and the testimonial value of humanitarian actions bring these features close to the role that bioethics ought to adopt in the issue of neglected diseases.

Celebrations and negative views on humanitarian actions are based on diverse ideologies; what remains relevant is the almost exclusive reliance on symptomatic proximal relief that cannot address the pathologies of power, at times even mitigating the sting of their deleterious politics. Equally problematic is the relationship between humanitarianism and human rights, seen by some as a necessary convergence in an era of globalization, whereas others insist on keeping them apart.

## V. INCENTIVE-BASED PROPOSALS

To spurn R&D for NTDs, push/pull mechanisms have been proposed, especially to energize product-development partnerships (PDP). Push mechanisms support the initiation of research ventures –investment, subsidies, and protocol elaborations–; pull strategies refer to providing incentives for "development and manufacture", that is, making available the final product –advance market commitments, patent extensions, prizes and patent buyouts– (Callan and Gillespie 2007).

Pharmaceuticals for developing countries need to be "clinically effective, cheap to manufacture, stable during distribution and storage, and easy to administer to ensure wide usage…About half of the drugs being developed to treat neglected diseases fail some of these criteria" (Hopkins, Witty and Nwaka 2007, 167).

Vigorous R&D is an indispensable policy to find innovative medical and public health products to treat NTDs that lack adequate therapeutic and preventive tools. Available agents are often unsuitable for local needs: intravenous administration, repeated dosage, disturbing side effects, and tradition-inspired local aversions. Furthermore, injudicious use of available

134            *Miguel Kottow*

products causes the increased resistance of infectious organisms and vectors. Even if biomedical assistance is recognized as patchwork, it nevertheless is essential to treat affected individuals as well as the public health vulnerability of poor populations, and must continue its efforts at developing effective therapeutic and preventive agents, hopefully to be supported by more comprehensive socioeconomic measures (Gostin and Powers 2006).

An elaborate pull incentive for R&D is the proposal of a "priority-review voucher" based on five criteria: focus on neglected disease, receipt of approval by the FDA or the EMEA (European Agency for the Evaluation of Medicinal Products), clinical superiority, relinquishment of patent rights, and assured availability of a manufacturer.

The maze of published material might suggest that most problems concerning NTDs are on their way out, so that the term neglect no longer applies. Unfortunately, results do not support these expectations, nor do the commitments of some major players in the field: governments are withholding their financial support and the pharmaceutics industry, despite goodwill proclamations, persists in its predatory practices: market exclusivity secured by patents, high prices commanded by positions of monopoly, R&D focused on low-risk failures and high potential earnings.

## A. Advance Market Commitment

Advance Market Commitment (AMC) proposes the creation of government-provided funds to be "committed in advance to make payments to any firm that can produce and sell a qualifying drug or vaccine." Funders guarantee a substantial income to drug-producers who will refrain from patenting in return for a fixed price to be held beyond the exhaustion of the agreed upon fund. The AMC "can only be applied to a rather limited set of products: the most likely candidates are vaccines in late-stage development, since the technical characteristics of such products can be described relatively well at that stage" (Hollis 2008, 126). The AMC is a scheme for controlling prices at the distribution level, rather than

*Coping with Neglected Populations* 135

stimulating research, depending on the drug manufacturer's appraisal of the benefit/costs ratio of securing a limited income or preferring to patent and hope for unlimited revenues.

The AMC was received with interest by major stakeholders –low-income countries requiring vaccine programs, international and national governments, and major pharmaceutical firms– and was implemented as a pilot project for pneumococcal vaccines in 2009. First evaluations were encouraging at the initial stages of an ongoing 10-year agreement, and a more complete assessment is pending, it being too early for a definitive evaluation of this project and its eventual application to anything other than vaccines and pharmaceutical and health-unrelated commercial products.

In a similar line of multilateral alliance, the Global Alliance for Vaccines and Immunization Gavi –known as the GAVI Alliance or simply GAVI–, is a major public-private alliance launched in 2000, committed to fund healthcare systems, negotiate prices for vaccines, and "introduce specific market-shaping mechanisms", whatever that may mean.

## B. The Health Impact Fund

Commenting on the Ebola outbreak of 2014, and the neglect that had hindered developing a timely vaccine, Peter Singer wrote

> Pharmaceutical companies are not charities. If we want them to make vaccines and treatments that will help the poor in the developing countries, we need to find ways of giving them –and their shareholders– a return on their investment.
>
> One promising attempt to correct this imbalance is the proposal for a Health Impact Fund that Thomas Pogge, director of the Global Justice Program at Yale, and Aidan Hollis, an economist at the University of Calgary, launched seven years ago. (Singer 2015)

The most innovative policy to stimulate R&D for rare and neglected diseases comes from Thomas Pogge, a well-known philosopher who is outspoken about global injustice and imaginatively active in the creation and development of the Health Impact Fund (HIF). Arguably the most widely discussed proposal, the HIF elaborates on the idea that the pharmaceutical industry foregoes patenting and the lucrative advantages of high-pricing a new product that exclusively dominates the market, by preferring to register with the HIF and agreeing to sell its product at cost price. Government-financed HIF would pay the drug company in proportion to the product's "assessed global health impact". The greater the preventive or therapeutic value of the product, and the more people benefiting from its availability, accessibility and efficacy, the more lucrative it will be for the manufacturer. The HIF is to be financed by a pool of consenting governments contributing in accordance with their "relative wealth" (Ooms and Hammonds 2008).

The HIF is substantially more complicated in its efforts to stimulate both research and price-controlled distribution. Interestingly, Pogge presents ethical arguments to support the moral obligation of participating in an R&D regulating policy. There is, he argues, an implicit general agreement that positive human rights are as important and binding as securing "negative duties not to violate these rights", together with an obligation to redress historical inequities of colonization, imperialism, and exploitation. Furthermore, Pogge claims that actual "huge inequalities" tend to perpetuate themselves, as wealthier countries wield power to secure their privileges (Pogge 2008, 76; Pogge 2009).

The proposal recruits the support of an impressive roster of eminent scholars, with numerous publications highlighting its advantages, but also pointing to its weaknesses. Suggestions have been presented with the argument that "an expansion of Pogge's proposal for patent reform – whereby health-promoting activities in general are incentivised in a similar way– would provide a more comprehensive solution to the healthcare situation in developing countries" (Selgelid 2008, 134). The implementation of the HIF would require rather complicated logistics, one of its main drawbacks being that global health impacts are very difficult to assess and predict over time.

Even though based on an incentive scheme that would not reduce the pharma industry's profit scheme, Pogge's elaboration of the HIF is based on intricate ethical arguments supporting the wealthy countries' duty to assist the poor and needy.

# VI. ETHICS-BASED PROPOSALS

> Systems awareness and systems design are important for health professionals, but are not enough. They are enabling mechanisms only. It is the ethical dimension of individuals that is essential to a system's success. Ultimately, the secret of quality is love. (A. Donabedian's interview with F. Mullan (https://doi.org/10.1377/hlthaff.20.1.137)

There have been some positive developments in the quest for lower prices and increasing availability, mostly of vaccines and drugs against VIH and hepatitis: The Drugs for Neglected Diseases initiative (DNDI), the Medicine Patent Pool (MPP) and others, achieve some remarkable results, observed with optimistic encouragement by some groups, though others lament that developing countries continue to labor under patent-based models. R&D policies persistently show little concern for "so-called neglected diseases", and the pharmaceutical industry's unrelenting pursuance of profits based on high prices for essential drugs, and aggressive policies to ensure a market monopoly at the cost of the reduced availability of much needed medication do not abate. "Without fixing this broken system we will not reach the Sustainable Development Goal to ensure healthy lives and wellbeing for all, at all ages. 'Leave no one behind', the UN's slogan, will prove to be empty words" (Ploumen and Schippers 2017, 341).

A high official of the South African Government is quoted as stating: "When a model is science-centric, it loses its ability to actually reflect early on the ethical question" (Singer et al. 2007, 163).

138                      *Miguel Kottow*

# VII. Moral Duty to Assist

The well-known utilitarian bioethicist Peter Singer has advocated for many years the idea of moral obligations to "those beyond our borders". His argument is plausibly based on the assumption that suffering and deprivation unto death is bad and, secondly, that "if it is in our power to prevent something bad from happening, without thereby sacrificing anything of comparable importance, we ought, morally, to do it" (Singer 1972, 231).

The individual assistance to the needy, as proposed by Singer (1972) is plausible when the deprived are proximate, circumstances are propitious or at least not adverse, and assistance is within the helper's capabilities. Three decades later he elaborates, arguing that, given that inequalities and suffering in affluent societies are less grievous than famine and extreme poverty overseas, aid should preferably go to the distant. The amount to be contributed ought to include all surplus income beyond providing "our own" –parents, children, and eventually next of kin and neighbors– "with the necessities of life, and also their more important wants, and must allow them to feel loved and protected" (Singer 2004, 18).

Singer's duty to assist elaborates on two actively discussed premises: reducing harm by way of assistance is impartial to where the needy are. The anonymous distant needy are to be assisted in their plight with the same, if not more, energy than the proximate destitute whose needs may be less basic or easier to satisfy by diverse methods. Secondly, individual assistance should be provided by surplus income and wealth beyond what is necessary for the comfortable but not luxurious upkeep of oneself and one's dependents. Such a substantial counterintuitive position becomes inconceivable in societies bent on self-sustenance, self-protection and self-responsibility, where the distinction is blurred between seeking a good life and securing the future, lived in a liquid modernity that, according to Z. Bauman, causes uncertainty, insecurity and a lack of protection. Not to mention the ethical apathy of consumer societies.

Discussing the right to a decent minimum of healthcare, which he rejected even though believing there might be a social duty to deliver it, philosopher Alan Buchanan (1984) proposed that the wealthy ought to gracefully contribute to finance some basic healthcare issues. But, he added, donators might be forgetful or disinclined to be beneficent, so why not introduce "enforced beneficence"? In the final analysis, the determination of a decent minimum, the right to healthcare, and a duty to provide are matters of "collective choice" and "some fair procedure for reaching a social decision" that cannot provide a universal moral duty to assist as Singer proposes.

"Instant communications and swift transportation" strongly suggest that "From the moral point of view, the development of the world into a 'global village' has made an important, though still unrecognized, difference to our moral situation" (Singer 1972, 232). If so, 45 years later the situation of neglected populations ought to have changed.

African bioethics believes that international help is under a "moral obligation" when "large numbers of people suffer in horrible ways in one part of the world, particularly to the point of their lives being threatened" (Metz 2018, 233). It is remarkable that a deontological demand is voiced together with criticism that the suffering populations have failed to provide the support of African ethics of fraternity, solidarity, and communal relationships, in the face of Ebola outbreaks in particular, and their native neglected diseases in general.

The diversion of surplus income towards aid would "ensure that the consumer society, dependent as it is on people spending on trivia rather than giving to famine relief, would slow down and perhaps disappear entirely. There are good reasons why this would be desirable in itself" (Singer 1972, 241). Such a proposition is what the German language calls *Weltfremd*, translated into English as the paler "unworldly".

## VIII. THE DISTANT NEEDY

For the last three centuries, the nation-state has evolved as a political unity with determined, though often disputed, borders that enclose a population living in an established social order. Citizens are subject to a

140  *Miguel Kottow*

regime of rights and duties, administered by a government with the foremost task of providing protection from injury, harm and need – freedom from want–. Even a limited cosmopolitan perspective may well recognize that if nations strive to honor basic moral standards of decency and mutual assistance to those in need, there is hardly any reason why this ethical stand should not expand transnationally:

> We can take the idea of national responsibility seriously and still recognize substantial obligations toward the world's poor...We can establish international standards of decency that entail an obligation to provide support for those people whose lives are currently less than adequate by those standards.
> A just world, on this view, would be one in which the principle of national responsibility was given full play, and which would therefore exhibit considerable diversity (including diversity of living standards), but in which remedial responsibilities were also fully acknowledged, so that no one was condemned to live a life below the threshold of decency. (Miller 2004, 140)

If these words were heeded, the distant needy would cease to suffer neglect as they become recipients of "remedial responsibilities". Exhausted of living a distant and needy life, they have embarked on a massive drive for proximity by launching interminable waves of immigration to nations where they will be seen, and hopefully assisted. But uncontrolled immigration is creating its own problems of poverty, inequity and hostility, which should be a warning for the powerful to reassess their indifference to the plight of the distant and neglected needy. Even those nations and global economic empires that have gravely contributed to inequity and poverty by exploitation, neocolonialism and, at best, assistance no larger than a drop in the bucket and ineffective unless blended with empowerment, have not taken up the responsibility of the guilty.

> The Standard View holds that this is the problem of whether we have a stronger duty to aid strangers who are physically near to us just because they are physically near than we have to aid strangers who are not

## Coping with Neglected Populations

141

physically near (that is, who are far), all other things being equal. A Standard Claim concerning this problem is that to say distance is morally relevant implies that our duty to aid a near stranger would be stronger than our duty to aid a far one, given their equal need. (Kamm 2004, 59)

The ethical criteria for assistance are guided by the degree of need and suffering to be reduced, rather than taking into account proximity or distance.

The meeting point of the proverb "The squeaking wheel gets the grease" and G. Spivak's famous question "Can the Subaltern speak?" is situated in the midst of the neglected, voiceless and unable to make themselves heard, treated as a statistical reality to be considered on the assisting agent's terms. Assistance to the far away poor is based on the acceptance that a political drive to universal justice remains a utopia that history and actual global affairs have no real intention to pursue. The economic drive of dominant capitalism and globalization will never have any serious intention of striving for a decent minimum. Headway for reducing poverty and neglect is mainly achieved by market economies implanted on a socialist base, as occurs in China, which has managed to substantially lessen poverty in a potent economy that does not shy away from maintaining severe income inequality. Granted that the international economic order is indifferent to the harmful inequities it causes and sustains, no effective global assistance to the poor can reasonably be expected.

The world has been downsized by the explosive growth of communications and the enormous flow of migrants, dulling the proximal/distal polarity, preferring the distinction between empowerment/disempowerment, outspoken/voiceless, inclusion/exclusion, recognized/neglected, and adhering to Foucault's distinction of modern biopower as the power to make live and let die. The present state of world affairs makes assistance to the distant needy as unreal as the quest for global justice.

*Chapter 8*

# BIOETHICS AND NEGLECTED DISEASES

## I. INTRODUCING BIOETHICS

As biotechnology and biomedicine are actively researching and proceeding to interfere with the human body's genetic and "normal" functionality, ethics has shown its holistic preoccupation by expanding into the perspective of an "ethics of the whole living world –human beings, animals and plants included", as practices in many non-Western cultures, and vividly professed by Albert Schweitzer (1875-1965) in his "Reverence for life".

The protestant theologian Fritz Jahr (1895-1953) coined the term *Bio-Ethik* in the late 1920s, publishing his views in the reputed journal *Kosmos*, where he presented a categorical Bio-Ethical Imperative based on Kant: "Respect every living being, including animals, as an end in itself and treat it, if possible, as such!" His work was rediscovered by H-M. Sass (2007), long after the American oncological researcher Van Renselaer Potter had claimed the paternity of "the term *Bioethics* in order to emphasize the two most important ingredients for achieving the new wisdom so desperately needed for humanity to survive: 'biological knowledge and human values'" (Potter 1971, 2). At the same time, André Hellegers came up with the name "bioethics" when creating and directing the Kennedy Institute of Ethics. Hellegers was centered on the practice of medicine and concern for

144                          *Miguel Kottow*

the underprivileged, as Reich comments: "The two ethical problems that haunted Hellegers were the worldwide disequilibrium between the powerful and the powerless, and the danger of exploitation of humans" (Reich 1995, 26). And yet, his institution's view was more restrictive "when Georgetown took the term 'bioethics' in the narrower direction of what one Georgetown scholar called a 'revitalized study of medical ethics,' expanded somewhat beyond the 'problems of physicians'" (p. 20).

The canonical definition presented in the *Encyclopedia of Bioethics* refers to the discipline as "the systematic study of the moral dimensions – including moral vision, decisions, conduct, and policies– of the life sciences and healthcare, employing a variety of ethical methodologies in an interdisciplinary setting." This comprehensive but undetermined description opened the doors to uncountable interpretations, often blurring the distinction between philosophical ethics and its practice-oriented application "as a study of morality as it concerns issues dealing with the biological issues and facts concerning ourselves, and our close relatives, for example, almost any non-human animal that is sentient" (Dittmer 2010, unnumbered).

By its nature as an applied ethics, bioethics needed to deal with the fact that different creeds would dismiss certain acts as contrary to human nature –abortion, euthanasia–. A variety of convictions had to deal with genetics and neuroscience filled with promises transforming and enhancing certain functional features of human beings that would either make them more apt to flourish or, to the contrary, negatively alter the moral substance of programmed autonomy (R. Dworkin). Post-human creatures would eliminate discrimination (Haraway), while eugenics was bound to harm the anthropological nature of the human (Habermas). No fundamental agreement could be construed on the basis of opposing views on human nature, to develop universally valid ethical maxims required by the quest for global ethics, condemning bioethics to endless strife and divisive biopolitical decisions.

From its inception, bioethics has been a philosopher's turf, heavy on theory and fairly poor on fulfilling its role as an applied or practical discipline initially called upon to help resolve the quandaries of patients

## Bioethics and Neglected Diseases

facing an increasingly sophisticated and science-based medical practice. Mounting theoretical interest was progressively invested in public health issues, biomedical research, and ecology, furthering a mélange between traditional matters of ethics and specific bioethics issues, the voice of common morality, the claims of experts, as well as the presence of self-appointed representatives of diverse ideologies. Academia began to churn out enormous numbers of articles and books on bioethics, supported by the creation of printed material strongly endorsed by avid publishing companies marketing journals, text books, book series and long-winded comprehensive and encyclopedic work steeped in scholastic rhetoric yet poorly attuned to social problems concerning health, disease, medical care, and human endeavors steering towards injustice and catastrophe in the wake of mounting healthcare disparities and neglect.

Leading publications tend to show a slight distinction between ethics and bioethics, referring to clinical bioethics as medical ethics, or giving a general description devoid of distinctive specificity when presenting bioethics as a "branch of ethics that investigates problems arising from medicine and biological innovations" (Churchill 1999, 253). The difference between the descriptive and normative inclinations of ethics as part of philosophical reflection, and bioethics as an applied form of propositional ethics focused on actual decision requiring problems of interpersonal and social relations, is eroded and completely lost if professional ethics get mixed with bioethical deliberation. Professional ethics have their normative expression in codes of ethics, whereas bioethics is, or should be, a continuous search for coherence and fairness.

The canonical early-bird textbook on bioethics –though ambiguously titled *Principles of Biomedical Ethics*– presented the so-called mantra of principlism –autonomy, beneficence, non-maleficence and justice–, eventually downgraded to *prima facie* principles that in practice have to be specified and balanced. European scholars developed their own brand of "bioethics and biolaw" principles: vulnerability, dignity, integrity and autonomy, giving priority to vulnerability.

Principlism has been found wanting, given that it reflects individual values, caters to Western worldviews, and is burdened by excessive

146                                    *Miguel Kottow*

academicism that ignores the quandaries and uncertainties at the social and public health levels. The first inkling that bioethics was ill-equipped to deal systematically with its diverse areas of competency became visible at the turn of the millennium with the emergence of public health bioethics, and the awkwardness of applying individual ethical principles to communities and populations.

> Bioethics is constructed in such a way as to ignore the role of social and cultural factors, partly because since it champions an 'ideal of universal ethical principles', such variations are regarded as 'epiphenomena' and unimportant. But beyond that, bioethics is wary about the 'invocation' of social and cultural factors since they are seen to lead towards 'local meanings' and thence to moral relativism and potential disaster. (Hedgecoe 2004, 125)
>
> It seems as if bioethicists have tended to provide broad but 'thin' reviews of potential ethical issues that stay within the boundaries of ethical discourse set by academic and industry scientists. They also have tended to avoid putting forward arguments for or against particular ethical positions. (Hedgecoe 2010, 176)

Initial efforts were devoted to a top-down strategy based on generally acceptable principles –principlism, maxims, and canonical casuistry– or paradigmatic cases –neo-casuistry–. In an age of secularity, many denied that ethics could rely on any universally acceptable maxims, preferring a bottom-up approach that studied situations, cases, and precedents. As is usual, extreme positions have relented to give an eclectic mixture that goes under the name of "coherentism": a mix of empirical evidence, theoretical basics, and deliberative elaboration (Beauchamp 2003).

Mainstream bioethics became institutionally established, giving rise to pre-graduate curricula, the post-graduate formation of "experts", the establishment commissions and committees, and the "self-congratulatory listing of *Core Competencies*" (Churchill 1999, 263), contributing to an unimaginative, stultifying, hair-splitting discourse: "An[other] issue germane to the social purpose of bioethics arises not from dealing with

*Bioethics and Neglected Diseases* 147

problems in the wrong way but from dealing with the wrong problems" (Ibid., 265).

Disputes on the subject remain endless as bioethics increasingly diverges from the concerns of its founders, splitting into clinical, biomedical, public health and ecological branches and subdivisions, with a strong tendency to focus on medical practice and biomedical research: "Medical bioethics, the mainstream of professional bioethics, has focused primarily on evaluating biomedical solutions to individual human disease and suffering at both disciplinary and institutional human levels of organization" (Beaver and Whitehouse 2017, 229).

> Bioethics...primary goal was to work for a more compassionate, less technocratic medical practice. These days that goal seems to be shifting. More and more often we hear from bioethicists who are not just pro-technology but much more fervently pro-technology than the public at large: bioethicists who consult for biotech firms, who work for pharma-funded bioethics centers, who write pro-industry articles, who not only think that pharma and biotech have the solution to our medical problems but that they have the solution to our social problems too. These writers exhibit the same kind of breathless enthusiasm for biotechnology that others have for, say, the computer revolution, or globalization. These are bioethicists for the wired generation. They genuinely believe that we can build a better society by building better people. (Elliott 2005, 21)

As concerns this book, bioethics took at least three turns that have deviated from recognition and concern for the problems of neglected diseases: the predominantly benevolent attention to technoscience, the concept of sustainability in its relations to future generations without having secured attention to unmet current needs (see Chapter 1-V), and the theoretical emphasis on global bioethics. Although it would seem counterintuitive to disparage matters so enthusiastically pursued by academia and the media, there can be little doubt and sufficient empirical evidence that inconsistencies in these areas are detrimental to an enlightened concern for neglected issues.

decades ago. Even though early efforts believed that the four principles could be applied to social health problems, it soon became apparent that population health requires its own, non-individualistic brand of bioethics, considering that what benefits a community may well be detrimental to individuals unwilling to sacrifice autonomy for the sake of promoting the public weal. The traditional view that public health is a matter of governmental responsibility has been weakened by the development of a "new public health".

> While new public health authorities and agencies continue to adopt overtly coercive strategies such as quarantine, isolation and enforced medical treatment when they seem required and most justified (such as in the face of a serious epidemic of infectious disease), they are equally, if not more, reliant upon the use of strategies that position citizens as acting of their own free will and in their own interests to protect their own health. (Petersen and Lupton 2000, 174)
>
> A strong emphasis on the ethic of self-care would seem to be directly at odds with the stated ideals in the new public health of nurturing social support, redressing inequality, and creating a tolerant democratic polity. (Ibid., 176)

Needless to say, this current approach to individual self-responsibility in healthcare and disease prevention is severely harmful to the poorer segments of unequal societies.

The major expansion of bioethics has failed to give enough thought to the fact that "non-Western" countries possibly have other bioethical concerns than those entertained by Anglophone scholars. No wonder that bioethics neglects issues like the industrial expropriation of natural medicine's traditions and therapeutic substances in low-income countries, the inappropriate discourses on social environments steeped in healthcare inequities, or the drive to utilitarian self-interested research ethics in poor nations expected to conform to lenient pragmatic ethics as compared to home-grown aspirational requirements (Macklin 2004).

The technocentric about-turn of mainstream bioethics disqualifies any attempt to engage the discipline in the problems of neglected diseases and

*Bioethics and Neglected Diseases*     151

rare afflictions, which to a great extent are caused and perpetuated by the unrelenting profit-oriented managed biomedical and pharmaceutical practices. And yet, new efforts are urgently needed to show that the forces of disparity and neglect are deploying new strategies in the wrong direction.

## III. GLOBAL BIOETHICS

In recent decades many voices have raised criticism of the scholarly engagement of bioethics finessing and celebrating sophisticated biotechnology, instead of moving on to global or holistic concerns. Global ethics/bioethics approaches differ in their preferred targets, ranging from sustainable growth, proactive respect for human rights and "freedom from want" –F. D. Roosevelt–, universal social security "from cradle to grave" – Beveridge–, the reduction of inequalities, the drive towards global justice, and the eradication of poverty. Some proposals are specifically aimed at one target to be universally achieved: "Meanwhile, the humanitarian imperative for the world to focus more on diseases of the poor in reaping the benefits of new genomics has still not been sufficiently addressed" (Yuthavong 2013, 122). Others stress the magnitude of globalization's negative effects, and the urgency of remedial actions: "Bioethics is taking into account more and more the effects of globalization, focusing on the forgotten, the invisible and the ignored billions of people who are powerless and voiceless, and lack basic healthcare" (ten Have 2015, 148).

Bioethics is correctly focused when denouncing the massive negative effects of globalization, yet it gets entrapped in a discourse of universal values, the meaning of which varies in diverse cultures. Individual autonomy, for example, is highly valued in Western culture, but of considerably less interest in Asian countries where each person is part of a family, tradition and nature. Furthermore, bioethics preaches justice, yet "is part and parcel of the injustices of the Western health care industry" (Chattopadhyay and De Vries 2008, 4).

# 152                          *Miguel Kottow*

Global bioethics rushed into the promising field of creating journals, publishing books, and making believe that their efforts would lead to a better and more just world by cancelling the insufficiencies of the past, and tackling all the problems that loom over humanity: depletion, pollution, inequity, marginalization, discrimination, exploitation, unprotected ageing, violence, and unfettered technoscientific expansion. Most of the scourges listed are caused by neoliberal globalization that cannot be effectively addressed by a global ethics incapable of becoming convincingly instrumental. In its ambitious flight, global bioethics became oblivious to the concerns of humanitarian values, to the lack of a bridge to the future – Potter–, and the faulty and declining mutual respect between science and the humanities –Snow–.

The initially negative reception of genetically modified food has taught scientists, assisted by sociologists, to develop and publicize their own ethical discourse before they plan to introduce novel biological products. Social studies show that bioethicists are technophiles generally supporting innovations with arguments that lack timeliness and originality, or are subservient to corporative campaigns supporting public expectations of marketable innovations "protected" by precautionary ethics, erroneously assuring public opinion that favorable benefits/risks ratios are carefully and continuously being researched.

The main problem that global ethics faces is inequality creating worldwide injustice, and the answer near at hand is to plead for distributive justice.

> Discussions of global justice in contemporary political philosophy tend to take place within a distributive framework, asking which inequalities between people living in the global North and those living in the global South are unacceptable and require redress. The distributive – or, more accurately redistributive– paradigm thus steers us towards solutions to injustice that center on a more equitable sharing of the earth's resources and opportunities. Such a redistribution is of course essential from the standpoint of a normative commitment to greater global justice. (Deveaux and Walker 2013, 111)

*Bioethics and Neglected Diseases*     153

Global ethicists try to ignore that neoliberal globalization has become the dominant, and arguably the only viable political strategy after socialism crumbled or negotiated its entry into the market economy. The downfall of capitalism as Marx hopefully predicted is not in view, quite to the contrary, the system has shown enormous suppleness when in crisis. There are potent reasons to believe the irreversibility of this trend, and its resilience when suffering economic backlashes that would seem to weaken the system's foundations finally allows it to resurface unscathed and even strengthened. According to the economist Vito Tanzi, the expansion of globalization will include strategies that will decrease national tax revenues, thus exacerbating social and international inequality, and deepening the plight of the underprivileged.

Healthcare problems are inextricably related to inequity, and neglected diseases are prominent but unattended issues that appear to be caused, or at least exacerbated, by disparities in medical services. Global bioethics is too wide-meshed to catch the slippery strategies of injustice and neglect; global perspectives, submerged in the broad, but ineffectual, presentation of healthcare disparities, inequalities, and calls for global solidarity, ignore specific issues urgently in need of attention.

The pertinence of global bioethics is usually illustrated by the reaction against pandemic infectious diseases, most notably counteracting the worldwide spread of HIV/AIDS. As the worldwide infection killed millions, responses were shown to contain damage in richer countries rather than broaching global solutions, beyond a general discomfort with unethical research, discriminatory public health policies, obstacles and the distribution of effective medication, high-pricing, unequal access, international conflicts concerning patents and compulsory licensing.

A still less praiseworthy reaction occurred during the $H_1N_1$ flu pandemic of 2009, which was shrouded in controversy and claims that the WHO had declared a false pandemic advised by experts who turned out to have financial ties with drug companies producing antivirals and vaccines (Godlee 2010). Many countries bought vaccines in excess, whereas others did not heed the WHO's warnings and fared quite well. The least that

154 *Miguel Kottow*

global solutions require is solidarity and fairness; lacking these basic ethical ingredients, global bioethics becomes a fatuous proposition.

Public health ethics, the currency of half-baked talk about sustainable growth, care for future generations, and artificial moral enhancement, and eugenics, cyborgs, and post-humans–, struggle with bioethics principles applied to individuals, stumbling on their way towards bioethics for collectives with the goal of installing some sort of global bioethics.

Not a definition, but an interesting overview claims, that "in some settings, life expectancy has declined as a result of HIV, tuberculosis, malaria, malnutrition, and violence", concluding that

> Bioethicists need to more competently address the complexities of global health; they need to expand their frame of analysis from wealthy societies and engage ethical issues in a globalizing world of extreme inequalities in wealth and health. (Turner 2007, 231)

# IV. ETHICS OF BIOETHICS

The queen of applied ethics was being questioned as to the scope and form of developing a discipline that basks in academic self-importance, but fails to integrate with social practices and cultural values destabilized by the neoliberal merchandizing of basic goods and essential services degraded to commodities. The Greco-French philosopher Cornelius Castoriadis asked many years ago whether principles in bioethics only became universal above a certain level of per capita gross domestic product.

Exploring the discipline's epistemological methods bioethicists stressed the importance of deliberation in a contemporaneous realm of multiculturality and pluralism, aimed at reaching consensus on valid principles and practical solutions to dilemmatic problems in clinical medicine and biomedical research and, more obliquely, addressing issues of ecological dimensions, where policies were enacted by a system unable

## Bioethics and Neglected Diseases

155

to be accountable to the anonymous mass of people that were being affected by public health actions.

Paul Farmer criticizes bioethics for its preferred focus on issues pertaining to industrialized nations while giving little attention to the social and medical problems of the poor: "What does bioethics have to say about this, the leading ethical question of our times? Almost nothing. Conventional medical ethics does a good job of erasing such obscene disparities, for at least four reasons":

> Ethics draws strength form experience-distant disciplines...medical ethics has been to a large extent a phenomenon of industrialized nations...medical ethics and bioethics...experts have dominated public discourse...in the hospital we are asked to address the 'quandary of ethics' of individual patients. (Farmer 2009, Loc. 2954, Kindle ed.)

Farmer's grievance against bioethics' lack of social relevance is also confirmed by the meagerness of sustained concern for "the disgrace of a health-system that rations access by ability to pay" (Churchill 1999, 266).

In the present context, consideration must be given to at least two fault lines: mainstream bioethics is guilty of a sustained penchant in favor of the technoscientific expansions of biomedicine, and of an alarming increase in conflicts of interest between honest scholarship and material privileges. Both tendencies impinge directly on healthcare disparities and neglect.

Academia has gained in exposure and sophistication, fostering the growth of experts in bioethics known as bioethicists who often act as stakeholders on the payroll of biomedical institutions –the pharmaceutical industry, genetics R&D– taking refuge in a widespread tolerance of conflicts of interests, the delivery of goods to a ravenous publishing industry, and microscopic devotion to intellectual minutiae.

> It is possible to describe bioethics as a commodity in a market economy, and if the right social and institutional structures are developed, that is exactly what it will become. But would that development be good for anyone other than bioethics entrepreneurs? (Elliott 2002).

# 156 *Miguel Kottow*

The philosopher Carl Elliott has been very outspoken on the matter of the unwholesome position of bioethical advisers accepting lucrative positions in the pharmaceutical industry.

> The thing that worries me about bioethicists and these technologies is that so many of the innovations are driven by marketing. And with a handful of exceptions, bioethicists have generally not paid that issue any attention at all. The drug industry has just gotten more and more powerful over the last decade, and bioethicists don't seem to be worried at all. In fact, a lot of bioethicists are now on the drug-industry payroll themselves.

Asked how this works, Elliott expands in an interview with The Atlantic:

> Well, there are a few things. There are a handful of bioethics centers that actually solicit funding from the drug industry, and there are a handful of independent bioethics think tanks that also get drug-industry funding. Bioethicists also work as consultants for the drug and biotech industries, serving as ethics advisors, ethics consultants, and members of ethics advisory boards. And there has been a move over the past decade, particularly over the past five to seven years or so, where most of the drug-industry research money that was going to universities is beginning to go to private contract research organizations. And with private businesses rather than universities getting the money and carrying out the research, there's a niche for a new kind of ethics review board—so-called 'non-institutional review boards.' That's another way for bioethicists to get in on the industry money. (Elliott 2003)

Misconduct and ethical transgressions are notably related to flourishing enterprises like managed care, the drug industry, for profit research organizations, and marketable genetics. Overall, bioethics has been a tolerant observer, at times putting its "expertise" on the market.

> Bioethicists now consult in hospitals, testify as expert witnesses in court, write regulatory policies, appear as expert commentators in the media, and fill positions of bureaucratic authority in pharmaceutical

## Bioethics and Neglected Diseases 157

companies, professional bodies, and government organizations... Bioethicists are treated as experts whose judgments on ethical matters must be solicited, quoted, paid for, deferred to, and perhaps occasionally refuted or criticized, but in all cases, given the proper respect. (Elliott 2007, 44).

Conflicts of interests between the research community and scientific journals have reached levels that concern UNESCO and many governments, despite initiatives to curb unethical scientific practices. Prime examples of confusion are conflicts of interests, involving skewing statistics or giving dishonest moral advice for financial gain, which really are ethical transgressions. Research ethics deals with both blatant ethical transgressions –plagiarism–, and bioethical issues –nondisclosure of placebo control groups–. The participation and toleration of these practices by bioethics are not surprising but ethically all the more condemnable because bioethicists are expected to regulate the ethics of research through IRBs, editorial assistance, consultation, teaching and training. The reliability and influence of bioethics require doing ethics, not just talking about them.

As long as bioethics sells its expertise and accepts paid employment in pharmaceutical industries and genetic enterprises it is sleeping with the enemy, and cannot be expected to make significant contributions to the ethical value issues involved in the problems of neglected diseases.

The time was ripe to generate new ways of approaching the implications and consequences of leading-edge biomedical research explosively being developed by genetics. Bioethics was not up to the task, becoming overtly criticized for its "advocacy" and "facilitation" of science and technology. The Human Genome Project (1990-2003) declared it would devote 5% of its research budget to a newly conceived program called ELSI: Ethical, Legal and Social Implications of life sciences research, shortly to be followed by its European equivalent ELSA. These programs took it upon themselves to increase public participation and interdisciplinary interaction –including the social sciences and the

158                *Miguel Kottow*

humanities– with the aim of expanding the diverse perspectives and amplifying the presence of actual and future stakeholders.

> Society should have a say in how the money is invested, i.e., transmutated into knowledge (which, hopefully, and eventually, can be transmutated back into money once again, through a process which is now often referred to as 'valorisation'). Moreover, society will function as the future *consumer* of the scientific knowledge thus produced, and as the *future* for new technological devices. (Zwart, Landeweerd and van Rooij 2014, 20)

## V. EXPLORING BIOETHICAL RESPONSES

Bioethics is a discipline that reflects upon man-made actions that have durable, often irreversible effects on values pertaining to life processes and transformations of nature. In a first approach, it would appear that the issue of neglected diseases is a political and economic one; yet, as first argued by Aristotle, politics is based on ethics, and even the most liberal economics are to be legitimated by moral consideration, as Adam Smith taught. Bioethics needs to be involved in setting the fundamental political actions or omissions in public health matters, and also in assisting fair and decent market functioning, including State surveillance, and encouraging care and protection for the destitute.

Bioethics is misconceived as a normative discipline when ignoring that its main focus is to deliberate and serve in an advisory capacity in specific clinical settings, and by bringing clarity and enlightenment to problematic and dilemmatic situations in biomedical and allied disciplines. Its mission is to participate in debates bringing to the fore all pertinent values that need to be considered, at best supplying a recommendation but not a norm. Lacking expert knowledge and social power, bioethics is poorly equipped to be normative, and inherently inconsistent when trying to impose principles or dogmas.

Bioethics is out of its league where economic considerations restrict resources that leave the weak and underprivileged unprotected. When insufficient public health or medical resources require rationing, bioethics has been willing to participate in debates about QALY, DALY or other forms of redistributing scarce resources, though its conclusions have often been criticized as occurs, for example, with Daniel Callahan's suggestions for a sustainable medicine that will reduce medical care for the elderly to a sufficient minimum. Rationing schemes should not belong to the realm of bioethics, for there is no justifiable criterion to draw a line between those included and those excluded.

Bioethics has been moderately successful in its efforts to reduce overt paternalism in medical practice, although fair participation is curbed by managed care, the financial restraints of national healthcare services, and residual authoritarianism that too often flares up. In other fields of life sciences, notably biomedical research and public health, bioethics has been even less influential.

Bioethics needs to improve the scarce and weak empowerment it has gained by institutionalizing committees and commissions. Bioethicists claim to legitimize its discourse by appealing to common morality, but they are countered by sociologists' demand for more empirical work for an accurate bottom-up understanding of public beliefs and social practices. Even the interplay between inductive and deductive propositions has proven unable to reach beyond theoretical disquisitions with limited practical clout. A hardly surprising state of affairs, considering that bioethics was initially the turf of theologians and philosophers engaged in analytic philosophy with a "commitment to universal theories" (Evans 2006, 225). Excessive and uncommitted theorizing has been calling for trouble, for bioethics is expected to perform as a practical ethics assisting healthcare practitioners in taking clinical decisions, improving research ethics and counseling on public health issues (Table 7.1.). Agreement and consensus have been hard to come by, positions often splitting into a philosophical camp strong on reflection but unaware of decision-making urgency, and a practical camp impatient with too much reasoning that delayed solutions to pressing problems.

# 160 *Miguel Kottow*

**Table 7.1. Suggested role for bioethics in neglected and rare diseases**

A. Upstream fieldwork
- Ethnographic bioethics
- Phenomenological fieldwork

B. Downstream inclusive participation in
- Research policies and planning
- Subject friendly bioethical research committees
- Host community friendly surveillance
- Decisive participation in patent and registration procedures

There have been calls for bioethics to adopt an activist role in the political arena or adhere to a militant position in social movements and discriminated groups. Feminism has been extremely successful in blending the theory of many disciplines including bioethics with strongly voiced social actions against gender discrimination, effectively demanding equality in all walks of life. Calls for reinforcement from bioethics to combat racism, to support and protect undocumented immigrants and discriminated ethnic minorities, should not remain unanswered.

> This also means spending less time explaining how awful things are to those who live them personally, or presenting purely technical or policy solutions that might work if only the powerful had the good will to undertake them and spending more time speaking among ourselves about *what are we going to do about the fact that things are bad and this is shored up by entrenched interests*: in other words, discussing our own agency. (Cox 2015, 46)

The attention of the sociologist Cox is directed to the cleft between academic and activist work, falling back on Gramsci's distinction between uncommitted traditional intellectuals, and the socially active organic intellectuals. Activist social movements mainly consider information they gain from everyday life and the political context, whereas academics tend to create endogamous knowledge that is served within their theoretical confines.

*Bioethics and Neglected Diseases* 161

Wherever bioethicists have done their field homework, it is important for their experience and knowledge to be shared. But when it comes to activism, the question is whether they do so *qua* bioethicists or simply as engaged citizens who join a social movement to aspire for differentiation without discrimination. Bioethics as a discipline must strive for solid foundations to address pressing public issues before launching, if at all, into the frays of activism. Credibility must be regained in order to avoid a further decline of the discipline, displaying a clear effort to disallow the bioethics community from sharing vested interests with big corporations.

## VI. UPSTREAM ETHNOGRAPHY IN BIOETHICS

The distinction between emic –participatory– and etic –observational– ethnographic research has been widely adopted by anthropological researchers, but has failed to touch the shores of bioethics. In fact, anthropology and bioethics have had only occasional encounters, mainly focused on specific issues such as the patient-physician relationship, medical care in Western biomedicine, child and elderly abuse, and decisions at the extremes of life –artificial reproduction, genetic diagnosis, and euthanasia–. Recent efforts based on the role of the place and situation of healthcare issues call for a reappraisal of the important roles of social capital, collective efficacy, communal organization, and empowerment of community residents as agents of change for improving local conditions that impact health: "research is needed to guide upstream approaches, including place-based interventions, which address contextual factors that shape major public health problems" (Amaro 2014, 964). Obviously, this agenda addresses upstream actions applied to firmly constituted communities, although the editorialist does briefly comment on "place-based" upstream research and intervention in low-income and minority communities. This is an interesting proposition when places are meant as territory with dwellers, not mere occupiers, bringing up the idea that neglected populations may be living in "a space of injustice and unfreedom" (Jennings 2015, 14), thus in part explaining the massive number of migrants in our times who, rather than being displaced persons, are human beings fleeing from the miseries of their home-space in search of safe and stable settlement but finding neither as they endlessly huddle in fragile refugee camps.

Even though multidisciplinary, bioethics has mainly developed along Eurocentric and Anglophonic pathways, with a strong tendency towards analytical and deductive thought best exemplified by the triumphal expansion of principlism, and the adherence to supposedly universally and culturally independent premises, as illustrated by UNESCO's Universal Declaration on Bioethics and Human Rights. Criticism of bioethics by social scientists has often been hostile, accusing bioethicists of being "armchair philosophers", "servants of established social and economic authorities", "creative narrators", and "show dogs". In defense of these and many other disparaging epithets, it has been claimed that such mudslinging is to be taken cautiously since it is itself not based on "careful empirical research"; but benignly shielding bioethics as becoming "considerably more multifaceted" is equally unsubstantiated by empirical evidence (Turner 2009).

Bioethicists are not ethnographers, nor are they anthropologists, but much can be gained by studying the work of medical anthropologists such as Kleinman, Good, Delvechio, Fassin and others, applying their methodology to get an internal view of the suffering and neglected poor as lived by affected individuals: to gain insight into the distant needy by a proximal approach of sharing and participating, whether it is understood as emic bioethics, a phenomenological approach or a perception-oriented view, as Sen describes the internal approach. This vivid account of the lived life of affected individuals is an indispensable complement to the external view of statistics, and the demand for accountability of measures and policies undertaken. The singular lived experience of being neglected and misrecognized needs to be ethnographically perceived to enliven the statistics insensitively feeding the view from above, and stress the urgency of relieving the plights of living human bodies.

# Bioethics and Neglected Diseases 163

The psychiatrist and medical anthropologist Arthur Kleinman has produced important work in the area of medical ethnography and the bridging of empirical findings with bioethical theory

> Empirical research can provide knowledge about local worlds of experience...knowledge that is useful, even essential, for bioethics. (Kleinman 1999, 71)

> The irrelevance of ethics can be seen when considering universal ethical formulations of justice and equity that do not begin with the local moral conditions of poor people, those experiencing the systematic injustice of higher disease rates and fewer health-care resources because of their positioning at the bottom of local social structures of power. (Ibid., 72)

> Bioethics requires both approaches: it must possess a method for accounting for local moral experience and a means of applying ethical deliberation. (Ibid., 73)

> Some of us have argued for such an ethnographic moment in policy and programs directed at social suffering. The obstacles to the realization of that moment are formidable; the language of policy is so powerfully controlled by economics, decision analysis, and legal procedure that it is difficult to pry open even a small space for ethnography. (Ibid., 89)

Beyond trying to bridge the traditional gap between theory and practice, ethnography is best suited to relate moral processes at the local level, and ethical discourse engaged by academics: "Ethnography is a method of knowledge production by which the ethnographer enters into the ordinary, everyday space of moral processes in a local world" Kleinman 1999, 77).

> To talk about universal ethical formulations of justice and equity, without beginning with the local moral condition of real people who experience the systematic injustices of higher rates of ill health and fewer health care resources owing to their position in local social structures of

164            *Miguel Kottow*

power is to make those formulations utopian and irrelevant to the local world. (Kleinman 2006, 271)

Ethnography is practiced in overlapping stages: 1) Self-knowledge of the observer's values and moral positioning; 2) Accurate and exhaustive descriptions of local values, morality, worldviews, the perception of, and engagement with, external social processes; and 3) Applying the knowledge gained to further interaction between local views and ethical action.

Ethnography contributes in different ways "to bioethics": (1) locating bioethical dilemmas in their social, political, economic, and ideological contexts; (2) explicating the beliefs and behaviors of involved individuals; (3) making tacit knowledge explicit; (4) highlighting differences between ideal norms and actual behaviors; (5) identifying previously unrecognized phenomena; and (6) generating new questions for research. More comparative and longitudinal ethnographic research can contribute to a better understanding of and responses to bioethical dilemmas, as do other quantitative and qualitative "methodologies" (Kon 2009).

The transcendental anthropological features of relating to others and managing to be-in-their own world are stifled and distorted in neglected communities, where integration into a stable and hospitable social milieu is too rudimentary and individual life conditions are too dire to advance the patterns of recognition required for the development of personal identity and integration into a public matrix of mutual rights and duties. Failure of these elements of recognition leads to pathologic states of misrecognition and neglect.

A major field of anthropological inquiry into ethical aspects of healthcare in non-Western cultures gives wind to cultural and ethical relativity, placing intricate problems onto analytical non-contextual bioethics and codified biomedical ethics. Ethnographic exploration at the individual level of people living in the midst of a neglected population helps to develop a narrative that bioethics could profitably explore to better understand what it means to be poor, marginalized beyond the familial and communal borders, unhinged from social processes, and eventually subject

## Bioethics and Neglected Diseases

165

to new and mostly baffling inclusion/exclusion criteria of assistance initiatives. By participating in the life-world of the neglected, directly observed ethnographic fieldwork may unveil basic misrecognitions and help to create a bridge leading to moral respect and acceptance (see Chapter 1 VIII-B). Serious bioethics must gain substance by going beyond statistics and third-person narratives, preferably embarking on a phenomenological exploration of singular experiences and firsthand knowledge of place and situation. The caring and responsive bioethicist will aim beyond anthropological ethnography in a cognitive process of committed participation and direct understanding. Also, the bioethicist experiencing the everyday life of the neglected persons will be in a position to assist in evaluating the availability and effective delivery of vaccines and other healthcare programs.

A bioethical ethnography of individuals anchored in neglected populations should help to avoid the dangers of advice-giving that risk being misled by the "Hawthorne effects" or self-fulfilling prophecies into which researchers fall when actually producing the findings they purport to describe.

Bioethics should cultivate a phenomenological perspective that listens to the first-person narratives of those living in misrecognized marginalization that needs to be corrected before equality in healthcare is undertaken. As long as neglected people remain as unrecognized human beings with a damaged identity, effective assistance will not reach them and public health programs will be patchy with only short-term benefits, if any at all. A bioethical view of the neglected person's suffering should help to create a virtuous circle of individual recognition, assistance, empowerment, and social recognition, as well as furthering empowerment in search of fairness in healthcare: "making *private* worlds *public*" as Pierre Bourdieu proposed.

> But the analyst will be able to make the most unavoidable intrusions acceptable only through a rewriting that reconciles two doubly contradictory goals. On the one hand, the discussion must provide all the elements necessary to analyze the interviewees' positions objectively and

166 *Miguel Kottow*

to understand their points of view, and it must accomplish this without setting up the objectivizing distance that reduces the individual to a specimen in a display case. (Bourdieu et al. 1999, 2)

Bioethics needs to work with the neglected population in an atmosphere of shared experiences and communication, realizing what a neglected existence means, and carrying the message to the neglecters.

# VII. DOWNSTREAM BIOETHICS: ADDRESSING THE NEGLECTERS

Bioethics should regain its original commitment to protect the underprivileged and regain trust in honest advocacy, decency and fairness; it will have to reinvent itself. Ties with corporative interests must be severed. The conservative view tolerating the *status quo* of the "worst humanitarian crisis since World War II" (J. Diehl in The Washington Post, 6/27/2017) ought to lead the agenda of reformed bioethics taking its place in issues that pertain to its core concerns with respect to healthcare neglect.

Increasingly, investigators are required to register their clinical studies in a publicly accessible database. This mandate has practical consequences to avoid unnecessary duplications, report negative studies, and keep track of the facts and reasons why trials are interrupted and discarded. Bioethical opinion should be included in these early phases of research planning, participating in the discussion of relevance and priority. If "me too" trials are presented while research for essential drugs is relegated, and research for rare diseases is put on hold, bioethics should press for its participation in the early stages of research policy settings, and provide public information about these processes, striving to be included as a stakeholder representing the voiceless, and not, as too often happens, defending its own vested interests aligned with those of profit-seeking healthcare entrepreneurial management, and delivering ancillary services to self-centered research and the knowledge market.

*Bioethics and Neglected Diseases* 167

The big industrial players will probably not rush to change their policy, but the *in situ* –impertinently interfering– presence of critical bioethics should help to discredit the esteem of the public image that the pharma corporations claim, by showing stains and lackluster that might, eventually, mollify their unlimited profit expectations and plant the seeds of social responsibility.

Research with animals, just as clinical trials with human beings, are mandated to be reviewed for approval by an *ad hoc* IRB or equivalent research ethics committee having jurisdiction at the sites chosen for trials. Off-shoring practices tend to take advantage of the delayed or less experienced review committees in low-income countries that are disparaged by adding insult to injury:

> It is evident that at least some of the problems that arise in attempting to provide adequate protection for the rights and welfare of human subjects can be traced to the way research is promoted by industry, with attractive financial inducements to governmental officials, developing country researchers and local institutions. A problem of a different sort is the deeply rooted, widespread corruption in developing countries. In both situations, there is little that well-intentioned researchers can do by themselves when they embark upon research aimed at improving the health conditions of populations in resource-poor countries. (Macklin 2004, 139)

Blaming the victim is a quick fix to close down the critical bioethics shop in biomedical research. In fact, review committees are overburdened by the amount of protocols they must look into, expediting work by becoming routinized experts on procedure –informed consent, confidentiality– and less concerned by questions of public relevance. Most pertinently, review committees should secure the delivery of local social value when sponsors and investigators initiate trial protocols in low-income research venues: "Results show that ethical review forms and guidelines overwhelmingly operate within a biomedical framework that rarely takes into account common CBPR [Community-based participatory research] experience" (Flicker et al. 2007, 478). Voices are emerging to

# 168 *Miguel Kottow*

require research in the LMIC to be responsive to local needs in terms of knowledge translatable into decision-making to address local healthcare problems (Wenner 2017).

To assure the local relevance of foreign sponsored pharmaceutical and biomedical research, a robust review process should be undergone especially focused on local consequences in terms of cognitive value, concrete benefits and specified risks. Such a procedure is to be carried out protecting the best interests of the weaker part –individuals, neglected populations, and low-income nations–, in an ethical way devoid of secondary interests. Cognitive solvency and honest evaluation ought to be at the core of trustable bioethics.

Bioethics' advocacy should protect the fragile and vulnerable against ambiguous international norms (Helsinki, CIOMS), allowing a margin of discretional interpretation that arbitrarily favors the powerful. When revising general norms and guidelines, past experience has repeatedly confirmed the decisive influence of vested corporative interest that time and again weakens suggestions to bolster the security and autonomy of research subjects and secure the needs and integrity of host communities.

IRBs ought to have a strong and predominant bioethical voice beyond the current endless minutiae concerning informed consent, certainly important issues that should nevertheless not overshadow the basic bioethical role of protecting subjects –fair assessment of risks, ancillary care, comprehensive insurance, and post-trial benefits– and host communities –local relevance and avoidance of abusive practices that are increasing healthcare disparities and neglect–.

Another level of pertinent influence occurs when applying for patent registration, especially if the dominant motivation is to protect the interests of the patent holder, not of the needy consumer: "Patent protection for chemical and pharmaceutical products is especially important compared with other industries because the actual manufacturing process is often easy to replicate and can be copied with a fraction of the investment of that required for the research and clinical testing" (Lehman 2003, 2). A non-co-opted bioethics ought to intervene at this level to insist that the maleficent circle of profit-oriented research, patents, high-priced products and

*Bioethics and Neglected Diseases* 169

unavailability should be tempered in favor of the suffering needy: rare diseases and neglected healthcare. As at the previous levels, bioethicists' intervention will begin by having little influence on the outcome, but it will allow them to publicly air pharmaceutical practices and help counter with well-founded criticism the industry's regrettable promotional efforts to appear as selfless guardians of medicine and with public health dedication to health and welfare.

The unflinching extreme profit orientation of managed medical services and the pharmaceutical industry is deeply embedded in the tangle of causes and effects of diseases affecting neglected populations, blue marble diseases and rare diseases. If bioethics intends to play a significant role in the matter of neglected diseases, it ought to recover its solo voice, maintaining a low profile in the repetitious discourses that lament the miseries of poverty and neglected diseases without gaining influence in the major political, economic and social processes that are involved. In the matter of neglected diseases, bioethics ought to focus on attacking the pharmaceutical industries' declared and unrelenting goal of securing profits at the cost of social responsibility. Its voice should be heard before neglectful corporative and public decisions are taken, and bioethics should strain for active and full participation in international documents that deal with all aspects of neglected populations, by forcefully displaying the firsthand phenomenological and contextual knowledge it has previously explored as to where and whom neglect hits.

*Chapter 9*

# GADFLY BIOETHICS

Healthcare neglect is no longer restricted to poor populations affected by infectious diseases, having become a global concern, as richer countries harbor pockets of poverty and neglect, and subject to a variety of factors – climate change, migrations, and economic issues–. The number of unprotected human beings is on the rise, as is the threat of endemic diseases exploding into devastating pandemics. Proclamations, programs and propositions to meet these challenges have been largely ineffectual, disarmed by the mushrooming of capitalism *sans* socialism: "The neo-liberal worldview is, thus, antagonistic to the recognition and protection of socio-economic rights at a foundational level" underpinned by "judicial globalization" (O'Connell 2011, 537). As ethics is colonized by instrumental reason, a plea is directed at bioethics to abandon aseptic academic filigree and conflicting interests, in favor of more robust critiques of corporative policies that are unjust and harmful.

## I. VISIBILITY OF NEGLECT

At the very least in terms of ecology, healthcare, social equity and security the actual state of the world is grievous, and has been declared so by many contemporaneous thinkers who deplore the damage being done by globalization, globalism, unfettered neoliberalism, and the growing polarization of the world's population into privileged and deprived, with a large intermediate area of competitive strugglers trying to "make a living" or at least survive. These are pessimistic views, unable to envision any form or way to alleviate man-made misery, but they are not nihilistic for they are motivated by a purpose: unveiling misfortunes is intended to create awareness that might at some point kindle the hope of mitigating despair and begin to dismantle it. Critical enlightenment counteracts the false sense of unsubstantiated holistic promises of improvement ushering in self-satisfied proclamations expected to take the sting out of the unseen problems of climate change, health inequities and neglected diseases.

Hans Jonas believed in a "heuristic of fear" that would help keep up unrelenting alarm and serve as a reminder of present and future threats of uncontrolled technoscientific expansion. In a similar vein, the heuristics of discontent and indignation displayed by critical theories pretend to do away with the harm-producing economics of unbound capital that grows inorganically. Contemporary societies are familiar with the phenomenon of social fear and concern, rarely even social panic, fueled by nuclear brinkmanship during the Cold War, and by the occasional flare-ups of international conflicts. Social restlessness is appealed to by forecasting ecological disasters that will drown, dry out or overheat the planet, or make it unlivable by massively poisoning waters and air, but they have rarely caused a general sensation of immediate threat.

Barring the menace of pandemics, healthcare problems do not create social unrest given that they only worry threatened individuals and distant populations, for the most serving as interesting quizzes for social scientists, philosophers and ethicists. Biomedical research efforts relentlessly pursue the discovery of marketable products, with little concern for social needs, delving in monopolistic practices, discriminatory distribution and constrained accessibility. Unfettered by neoliberal policies and practices, healthcare disparities continue to rise.

Initiatives to curb injustice and especially healthcare inequities have had only fragmented and temporary successes, yet the overall picture

*Gadfly Bioethics* 173

remains dire and is getting worse: The Global Burden of Disease (GBD) Study launched by *The Lancet* shows, according to a recent editorial "GBD 2017: a fragile world," (Nov. 10, 2018), that the disaggregation of major statistical findings unveils "how patchy progress is".

> Although NCDs will increasingly dominate the disease burden in most countries, in many lower-income countries communicable, maternal, neonatal, and nutritional diseases are forecast to still exact a high toll in 2040. (Blakely 2018, e14)

The generic application of Universal Healthcare (UHC) programs lacks precision and specificity to tackle NTDs, often with even detrimental effects –epidemic bouts due to insufficient prevention, resistant vectors and microorganisms caused by the injudicious use of disinfectants and antibiotics– The introduction of policies to curb infectious diseases has the paradoxical effect of increasing the prevalence of NCDs. A more durable success of technical assistance may eventually fail if economic globalization continues to expand and favor the few while leaving behind the many underprivileged and powerless to struggle against pervasive odds. Some regions have benefited from well-planned and adequately implemented programs, and these initiatives merit support and extension. All in all, health spending and development assistance need to be increased to benefit the world's poorest people, an oft-repeated conclusion confirming that the technical redistribution of resources is sparsely effective unless inspired by the ethical motivation of caring for the neglected.

## II. ETHICS UNDETERMINED

Ethical discourse has too often cast wide-angle images of utopias where justice prevails and communicative discourse legitimizes socially robust peace, Leviathan and its citizens comparing notes as they achieve a stable balance between the common weal and individual flourishing.

Ethical meanderings have lost clout after their criticism of the present and their hopes for a better future could no longer rely on a revolutionary political program.

Sad as it may sound, there is no supportive reason or insight to indicate that justice in general and healthcare equity in particular, are goals that humanity unerringly ought to strive for. Mankind dwells in the world making history, not following a predetermined destiny: neither Hegelian Absolute, Platonic Good nor transcendent Justice finds a place in modern secularity, where "no one can any longer believe in progress, in consensus, in transcendent values", according to the postmodern thinker J-F. Lyotard. Ethical values are caught in a musical chairs exercise tuned by the pragmatics of rational and useful enterprise that dictates the normative rightness of efficiency and the culpable wrongness of mistakes. Ethics no longer elaborates along the concepts of good and evil, for who is to say?

Perpetrators of violence and misdeeds affecting the integrity and identity of others rarely if ever express guilt, nor is remorse part of modern moral's tool kit. Quite to the contrary, pragmatism always looks ahead, neither looking back at past mistakes, nor down at possible stumbling blocks. If ethics has become unable to take an affirmative stance about what ought to be done, it should consider dissecting the origins of misfortune and culpability and guilt, the difficult but necessary unveiling of *ex post* responsibility, hopefully to evoke remorse and the intention of avoiding the repetition of harmful actions. Looking back at one's own misdeeds and the mistakes of others should help avoid them in the future, as Santayana repeatedly pointed out. Unless ethical accountability is delivered, morality flattens out into banality, as perhaps most clearly illustrated in Hannah Arendt's work on the banality of evil when reporting on Adolf Eichmann's trial in Israel. Impressed by the accused's imperviousness, she diagnosed him as unable to recognize evil, thus explaining, though in no way justifying his barbarous deeds, much to the outrage of Hans Jonas among others.

Accepting the banality of evil cuts a deep wound in the idea of ethics, and Arendt was wrong on two accounts. Firstly, banality could only result from insensitivity to account for grief and remorse caused by a totally

Gadfly Bioethics 175

disarrayed moral compass and, secondly, Eichmann's presumption that fulfilling the received orders of extermination freed him from ethical reflection was, as later demonstrated, a show of indifference manipulated to placate accusers and judges.

Evil is never banal, it needs to be recognized for what it is, in order to avoid its perpetuation. Before neglect can be erased, its harmful effects from the past merging into the present must be remorsefully depicted in their full gravity.

Recent history unleashes winds that swing social moods between remembering and forgetting. Genocides, totalitarian brutality, racial and sexual abuses, and many other massive atrocities are being carved into memory or drowned in forgetfulness, swinging between extremes activated by all sorts of passions available to episodic events, yet insensitive to chronic misery. Neglect is a cesspool, not a stream, a condition rather than an event that can be remembered or forgotten and that needs to be stirred into visibility.

Neglected diseases are no longer a categorical entity appropriately defined as unattended infectious conditions affecting the poor. Rather, they are a particular manifestation of a universal inequity in the access to required and existent medical and public health agents and procedures. The limitations or the absence of the human body's functionalities are progressively entrusted to individual responsibility in the wake of the decreasing support of social security, causing medicine to become a market-regulated service. Given that the lack of financial solvency means the loss of accessible medical and social protection, those who are or become unproductive will have no safety net to secure their basic needs: the poor, the elderly, the chronically diseased and the disabled, the unemployed and the outcasts are all condemned to deprivation and suffering. By any measure or value system, ethics and humanitarianism are being submerged by a limited number of people in the heated existential circularity of production and consumerism all too willing to ignore neglect.

As healthcare inequities also permeate richer countries, concerns aim at gaining some control over healthcare and medicalization that are damaging through overuse, though not as much as by underuse. New

176                               *Miguel Kottow*

schemes hoping for less inequity in healthcare matters without threatening high profits and economic power, as proposed in the Doha agreement, backfired in the TRIPs plus strategies and the expansion of depredatory FTAs. Interesting schemes suggest lowering prices and increasing the availability of essential preventive and therapeutic agents, in exchange for subsidizing the pharma industry's revenues so as not to threaten their profits or make it compulsory to abide by such plans. Programs like AMC or the HIF are confident of blueprinting win-win situations which in the end are efforts at redistribution that even if feasible will meet the unrelenting opposition of economic power. But winning battles, even winning a war, is never a win-win reality. It is, nevertheless, a commendable and admirable effort, the implementation of which should in no way be hindered by pessimistic critique.

## III. RESITUATING BIOETHICS

In his famous essay "How Medicine Saved the Life of Ethics" (1982), Stephen Toulmin remarked that ethics had dried up as an uninteresting branch of philosophy captured by analytic thought. Medicine was being seduced and co-opted by scientific evidence and technical proficiency that required prudential evaluation and the evaluation of intervention into processes of life, suffering and death matters. Toulmin proposed that ethics might be revitalized, taking up medical issues entrapped between anemic scientific evidence and humane, mutually respectful patient/physician relationships. This was a modest plea to infuse ethics with a meaningful agenda, inverting the traditional rescue that ethics saves the life of science by introducing values of social disciplines and the humanities.

> Whatever the future may bring, however, these 20 years of interaction with medicine, law, and the other professions have had a spectacular and irreversible effect on the methods and content of philosophical ethics. By reintroducing into ethical debate the vexed topics raised by *particular cases*, they have obliged philosophers to address

once again problems of *practical reasoning*, which had been on the sidelines for too long. In this sense, we may indeed say that during the last 20 years, medicine has 'saved the life of ethics', and that it has given back to ethics a seriousness and human relevance which it has seemed, at least in the writings of the interwar years –to have lost for good. (Toulmin, 1997, 34)

This article appeared in a comprehensive volume on bioethics published at a time when public health and bioethics had not yet met, and issues of healthcare inequity and neglect were yet to be introduced.

The neglect of equity in healthcare, the proclaimed but *de facto* ignored human right to health touted as "the economic, social and cultural right to a universal minimum standard of health to which all individuals are entitled", is a stark reality that is impervious to the founders of bioethics as an inspiration to save medicine from its obsession with science, and as a discipline commissioned to "save humanity" by the prudent use of practical reasoning.

Concepts are shifting and becoming increasingly polysemic, often ambiguous. Medical deontology used to imply the study of codes of medical ethics, later signified duty-bound medical practice as distinct from utilitarian or pragmatic medicine. It can be reasonably claimed that the obsolescent term "medical deontology" led to the unfolding of clinical bioethics, just as Potter´s global bioethics was intended to develop what he called "knowledge of how to use knowledge", a bridge between science and humanities, a revival of Aristotelian excellence in practical reasoning – *phronesis*.

It is inherent to the proper exercise of bioethics to avoid perspectives biased by participation in corporative interests. Quite to the contrary, bioethics should strive to denounce such interests as harming the vulnerable. In 2013, The UNESCO Chair in Bioethics of Haifa, Israel, hosted a comprehensive symposium on "The ethics of pharmaceutical industry influence in medicine". The obvious question is why there is only sporadic concern about "the ethics of pharmaceutical industry influence in bioethics". Ethics and bioethics are expected to decry flawed practices and

178                                    *Miguel Kottow*

be proficient at doling out blame and shame, but who controls the controllers?

UNESCO's publication "Global Ethics: What for?" (2015) presents the views of 30 highly prominent scholars and UNESCO-related past and present officials. From its blurb: "It is through bioethical discernment, with its complexity, cultural diversity, social differentiation and economic inequality that answers can be found, with our feet planted in local history but our sights set on the holistic horizon."

The track record of bioethics shows regrettable deviations from its original calling to protect the needy, the threatened and the forgotten in matters concerning health, disease, biomedical research and public health, and adaptation to environmental changes. The discipline is a frequent lamenter but a rare accuser. Unwilling to exercise unwelcome criticism, bioethics has to a great extent sailed in two non-aligned directions: academia and yesmanship. Its rhetoric is rarely scathing enough to point out misdeeds or take up the battle against the powerful. Its certainly desirable penchant for pluralistic deliberation has become an academic exercise in minutiae or untimely speculations that result in indecision, indetermination, discretional interpretations, recantations, and bland proclamations. True, activism is not its thing, but commitment ought to remain bioethics' core value. Bioethics is not an expertise, for moral experts would unethically claim truth and impose dogmas, decrying doubter and deniers, steering clear of being servile to the master Science.

The *raison d'être* of bioethics is intellectual honesty in deliberation, unbiased assistance in clinical, biomedical research and public health decision-making, striving to gain outreach to improve policies in matters of healthcare equity and related subjects.

Plato has Socrates saying: "I am that gadfly which God has attached to the state, and all day long and in all places am always fastening upon you, arousing and persuading and reproaching you."

Gadflies irritate and pester, they are unwilling to settle down and assimilate to *status quo* conditions. A residual hope for bioethics is to act as a steered gadfly, a moral drone, aiming at specific and identifiable sites that nourish the drama of biomedical and pharmaceutical endeavors

*Gadfly Bioethics* 179

flourishing in a market economy that is indifferent to social plights. The bioethical gadfly needs to enter the fortresses where biomedical priorities are set into policies, where corporative interests dominate over social need, profit outsmarts the affordability of basic wants, and concern is replaced by neglect.

# REFERENCES

Abrahamsson, S., and P. Simpson. 2011. "The Limits of the Body: Boundaries, Capacities, Thresholds." *Social and Cultural Geography* 12(4):331–338.

Affolder, R., I. Rizzo, C. Burgess, A. Bchir, and J. Lob-Levyt. 2007. "A Prescription for Drug Delivery." *Nature* 449(13):170–172.

Alkire, S., and J. E. Foster. 2008. "Counting and Multidimensional Poverty Measurements." *Journal of Public Economics.* Accessed September 5, 2018. http://www.un.org/en/ga/second/65/docs/foster.pdf.

Amaro, H. 2014. "The Action in Upstream Place-based Approaches for Achieving Population Health and Health Equity." *American Journal of Public Health* 104:964.

Andorno, R. 2007. "Global Bioethics at UNESCO: in Defence of the Universal Declaration on Bioethics and Human Rights." *Journal of Medical Ethics* 33:150–154.

Angell, M. 2005. *The Truth About the Drug Companies.* New York: Random House Trade.

Arendt, H. 1998. *The Human Condition.* Chicago: The University of Chicago Press.

Aronson, J. K. 2006. "Rare Diseases and Orphan Drugs." *British Journal of Clinical Pharmacology* 61(3):243–245.

Arras, J. D., and E. Fenton. 2009. *Hastings Center Report* 39: 27–38.

## References

Azam, M. 2016. *Intellectual Property and Public Health in the Developing World.* Cambridge, UK: Open Book Publishers.

Banerjee, A., A. Hollis, and T. Pogge. 2010. "The Health Impact Fund: Incentives for Improving Access to Medicines." *The Lancet* 375:166–169.

Baron, J. 2006. *Against Bioethics.* Cambridge Mass., London: The MIT Press.

Battin, M. P. 2003. "Bioethics." In *A Companion to Applied Ethics,* edited by R. G. Frey and C. H. Wellman, 295–312. Malden: Blackwell Publishing.

Bauman, Z. 2001. *Globalización. Las consecuencias humanas* [*Globalization. The Human Consequences*]. 2nd ed. México, Fondo de Cultura Económica. Translated from Bauman Z. 1998. Cambridge: Polity Press.

Bauman, Z. 2005. *Identity.* Cambridge: Polity Press.

Bauman, Z., and R. Raud. 2015. *Practices of Selfhood.* Cambridge: Polity Press. (Kindle version).

Bavisetty, S., W. Wayne, W. W. Grody, and S. Yazdani. 2013. "Emergence of Pediatric Rare Diseases." *Rare Diseases* 1:1. Accessed July 25, 2018. https://doi.org/10.4161/rdis.23579.

Beauchamp, T. L. 2003. "The Nature of Applied Ethics." In *A Companion to Applied Ethics,* edited by R. G. Frey and C. H. Wellman, 1–16. Malden: Blackwell Publishing.

Beaver, J., and P. J. Whitehouse. 2017. "The Ecosystem of Bioethics: Building Bridges to Public Health." *JAHR* 8/2 (16):227–243.

*Biodiversity.* 2010. Accessed June 1, 2018. http://biodiversity-corner. blogspot.com/p/intrinsic-value-of-biodiversity.html.

Benatar, S. R. 2005. "Moral Imagination: The Missing Component in Global Health." *PLOS Medicine.* Accessed June 23, 2018. doi: 101371/jotnal.pmed.0020400.

Bernhard, K. H., N. Houghton, and L. Teplitskaya. 2014. "Development Assistance for Neglected Tropical Diseases: Progress Since 2009." *International Health* 6(3):162–171.

## References 183

Blakely, T. 2018. "Major Stride in Forecasting Future Health." *The Lancet* 392 Nov. 10, (e14-e15).

Bourdieu, P., et al. 1999. *The Weight of the World*. Stanford: Stanford University Press.

Brandom, R. M. 2011. "The Structure of Desire and Recognition: Self-consciousness and Self-constitution." In *Recognition and social ontology, edited by A.* Laitinen and H. Ikäheimo, 40–66. Leiden: K. Brill NV.

Brown, W. 2006. "Power after Foucault." In *The Oxford Handbook of Political Theory*, edited by J. S. Dryzek, B. Honig, and A. Phillips, 65–84. Oxford: Oxford University Press.

Brunkhorst, H. *The Crisis of Legitimization in the World Society*. Accessed August 28, 2018. warwick.ac.uk/fac/soc/sociology/staff/robertfine/home/teachingmaterial/humanrights/pdfreadings/brunkhorst-the_crisis_of_legitimation_of_human_rights.pdf.

Buchanan, A. 1984. "The Right to a Decent Minimum of Health Care." *Philosophy and Public Affairs* 13(1):55–78.

Butler, D. 2007. "Lost in Translation." *Nature* 449(13):158–159.

Callahan, D. 1999. "Bioethics and Beyond." *Daedalus* 128(4):275–294.

Callan, B., and I. Gillespie. 2007. "The Path to New Medicines." *Nature* 449(13):164–165.

Casey, E. 2001. "The Ghost of Embodiment: Our Bodily Habitudes and Schemata." In *Body and Flesh*, edited by D. Welton. Malden: Blackwell Publishing.

Chattopadhyay, S., and R. De Vries. 2008. "Bioethical Concerns are Global, Bioethics is Western." *Eubios Journal of Asian International Bioethics* 18(4):106–109.

Churchill, L. 1999. "Are We Professionals? A Critical Look at the Social Role of Bioethicists." *Daedalus* 128(4):253–274.

Clarke, A. E. et al. 2003. "Biomedicalization: Technoscientific Transformations of Health, Illness, and the U.S. Biomedicine." *American Sociological Review* 68(2):161–194.

Clarke, J. T. R. 2006. "Is the Current Approach to Reviewing New Drugs Condemning the Victims of Rare Diseases to Death? A Call for a

## References

National Orphan Drug Review Policy." *Canadian Medical Association Journal* 174(2):189–190.

Conrad P. 2007. *The Medicalization of Society.* Baltimore: The Johns Hopkins University Press.

Correa, C. 2002 *Implications of the Doha Declaration on the TRIPS Agreement and Public Health.* Geneva: World Health Organization.

Cox, L. 2015. "Scholarships and Activism: A Social Movements Perspective." *Studies in Social Justice* 9(1):34–53.

Daniels, N., and J. Sabin. 1997. "Limits to Health Care: Fair Procedures, Democratic Deliberation, and the Legitimacy Problem for Insurers." *Philosophy and Public Affairs* 26:305–350.

Das, V. 1999. "Public Good, Ethics, and Everyday Life: Beyond the Boundaries of Bioethics." *Daedalus* 128(4):99–133.

Day, M. R., and P. Leahy-Warren. 2008. "Self-neglect 1: Recognising Features and Risk Factors. *Nursing Times* 104(24):26–27.

Dean, H. 2009. "Critiquing Capabilities: The Distractions of a Beguiling Concept." *Critical Social Policy* 29(2):261–273.

DeAngelis, C. D. 2016. "Big Pharma Profits and the Public Losses." *The Milbank Quarterly* 94(1):30–33.

Deveaux, M., and K. Walker. 2013. Introduction to *Journal of Global Ethics* 9(2):111–114.

Diependaele, L., J. Cockbain, and S. Sterckx. 2017. "Raising the Barriers to Access to Medicines in the Developing World –the Relentless Push for Data Exclusivity." *Developing World Bioethics* 17(1):11–21.

Dittmer, J. 2010. "Applied Ethics." *Internet Encyclopedia of Philosophy.* Accessed July 4, 2018. https://www.iep.utm.edu/ap-ethic/.

Doniec, K., R. Dall'Alba, and L. King. 2018. "Brazil's Health Catastrophe in the Making." *The Lancet* 392 (September 1):731.

Elliott, C. 2002. "Diary." *London Review of Books* 24(23):36–37.

Elliott, C. 2003. "The Pursuit of Happiness." *Atlantic Unbound* August 5, 2003. Accessed May 31, 2018. https://www.theatlantic.com/past/docs/unbound/interviews/int2003-08-05.htm.

Elliott, C. 2005. "Adventure! Comedy! Tragedy! Robots!" *Journal of Bioethical Inquiry* 2(1):18–23.

## References 185

Elliott, C. 2007. "The Tyranny of Expertise." In *The Ethics of Bioethics*, edited by L. A. Eckenwiler, and F. G. Cohn, 43–55. Baltimore: The Johns Hopkins University Press.

Esposito, R. 2009. *Tercera persona* [*Third person*].Buenos Aires: Amorrortu.

Esposito, R. 2010. "Flesh and Body in the Deconstruction of Christianity." *The Minnesota Review* 75:89–99.

Evans, J. H. 2006. "Between Technocracy and Democratic Legitimation: A Proposed Compromise Position for Common Morality Public Bioethics." *Journal of Medicine and Philosophy* 31:213–234.

Farmer, P. 2003. *Pathologies of Power: Health, Human Rights, and the New War on the Poor*. Berkeley, Los Angeles: University of California Press.

Fassin, D. 2007. "Humanitarianism as a Politics of Life." *Political Culture* 19(3):499–520.

Fellows, G. K., and A. Hollis. 2013. "Funding Innovations for Treatment for Rare Diseases: Adopting a Cost-based Yardstick Approach." *Orphanet Journal of Rare Diseases* 8:180–189.

Ferrarese, E. 2015. *Nancy Fraser and the Theory of Participatory Parity*. Books and Ideas, September 14. Unpaged.

Flicker, S., R. Travers, A. Guta, S. McDonald, and A. Meagh. 2007. "Ethical Dilemmas in Community-based Participatory Research: Recommendations for Institutional Review Boards." *Journal of Urban Health* 84(4):478–493.

Foreman, K. J., et al. 2018. "Forecasting Life Expectancy, Years of Life Lost, an All-cause and Cause-specific Mortality for 250 Causes of Death: Reference and Alternative Scenarios for 2016-40 for 195 Countries and Territories." *The Lancet* October 16. Accessed November 6, 2018. http://dx.doi.org/10.1016/S0140-6736(18)31694-5.

Frankfurt, H. 2015. *On Inequality*. Princeton: Princeton University Press (Kindle ed.).

Fraser, N. 2000. "Rethinking Recognition." *New Left Review* 3, May-June: 1–9.

Gardiner, M. E. 2004. "Wild publics and Grotesque Symposiums: Habermas and Bakhtin on Dialogue, Everyday Life and the Public Sphere." In *After Habermas: New Perspectives on the Public Sphere*, edited by N. Crossley and J. M. Roberts, 28–48. Oxford: Blackwell Publishing.

*Godlee, F. 2010.* "Conflicts of Interest and Pandemic Flu." *BMJ 340:c2947.*

Gostin, L. O., and M. Powers. 2006. "What Does Social Justice Require for The Public's Health? Public Health Ethics and Policy Imperatives." *Health Affairs* 25(4):1053–1060.

Graham, C. E. et al. 2014. "Current Trends in Biobanking for Rare Diseases: a Review. *Journal of Biorepository Science for Applied Medicine* 4(2):49–61.

*Gunson, D. 2009. "Solidarity and the Universal Declaration on Bioethics and Human Rights." Journal of Medicine and Philosophy* 34:241–260.

Haffner, M. E. 2016. "History of Orphan Drug Regulation –United States and Beyond." *Clinical Pharmacology and Therapeutics* 100(4):342–343.

Halpin, L., J. Savulescu, K. Talbot, M. Turner, and P. Talman. 2015. "Improving Access to Medicines: Empowering Patients in the Quest to Improve Treatment for Rare Lethal Diseases." *Journal of Medical Ethics* 41(12):987–979.

Harmon, S. H. E. 2006. "Solidarity: A (New) Ethic for Global Health Policy." *Health Care Analysis* 14:215–236.

Han, B-C. 2015. *The Burnout Society*. Stanford: Stanford University Press.

Hedgecoe, A. 2004. "Critical Bioethics: Beyond the Social Science Critique of Applied Ethics." *Bioethics* 18:120–143.

Hedgecoe, A. 2010. "Bioethics and the Reinforcement of Socio-technical Expectations." *Social Studies of Science* 40(2):163–186.

Hollis, A. 2008. "The Health Impact Fund: A Useful Supplement to the Patent System?" *Public Health Ethics* 1(2):124–133.

Homedes, N., and A. Ugalde. 2015. "Availability and Affordability of New Medicines in Latin American Countries where Pivotal Clinical Trials

## References 187

were Conducted." *Bulletin World Health Organization* 93(10):674–683.

Hopkins, A.L., M. J. Witty, and S. Nwaka. 2007. "Mission Possible." *Nature* 449(13):166–169.

Horton, R. 2012. "Offline: The Silence of the Organs." *The Lancet* 380, September 15.

Horton, R. 2018. "Offline: Frantz Fanon and the Origins of Global Health. *The Lancet* 392, September 1.

Hotez, P. 2007. "A New Voice for the Poor." *PloS Neglected Tropical Disease* 1(1):1.

Hotez, P. 2013. "NTDs V.2.0: 'Blue Marble Health' –Neglected Tropical Disease Control and Elimination in a Shifting Health Policy Landscape." *PLOS Neglected Tropical Diseases*, 7(11):1–7.

Hotez, P. 2018. "The Rise of Neglected Tropical Diseases in "New Texas"." *PloS Neglected Tropical Diseases* 12(1).

Hotez, P., A. Damania, and M. Naghavi. 2016. "Blue Marble Heath and the Global Burden of Disease Study 2013." *PLOS Neglected Tropical Diseases.* Accessed September 1, 2018. doi: 10.1371/journal. pntd.0004744.

Hotez., P., and S. J. Lee. 2017. "US Gulf Coast States: The Rise of Neglected Tropical Diseases in 'Flyover Nation'." *PLOS Neglected Tropical Diseases.* Accessed September 1, 2018. http://doiorg./ 10.1371/Journa.pntd.0005744.

Hottois. G., and J-N. Missa. (eds.). *Nouvelle encyclopédie de bioéthique* [*New encyclopedia of bioethics*]. Brussels: De Boeck & Larcer.

Huber, M., et al. 2011. "How Should We Define Health?" *British Medical Journal* 343:d4163.

Hunt, P. 2007. *Neglected Diseases: A Human Rights Analysis.* Geneva: WHO/TDR.

Huyard, C. 2013. "How did Uncommon Disorders become "Rare Diseases"? History of a Boundary Object." *Sociology of Health and Disease* 31(4):463–47.

Hyry, H. I., J. C. P. Roos, and T. M. Cox. 2015. "Orphan Drugs: Expensive Yet Necessary." *Quarterly Journal of Medicine* 108:269–272.

188          *References*

Hyry, H. I., A. D. Stern, T. M. Cox, and J. C. P. Roos. 2014. "Limits on Use of Health Economic Assessments for Rare Diseases." *Quarterly Journal of Medicine* 107:241–245.

Iser, M. 2013. "Recognition." *Stanford Encyclopedia of Philosophy.* Accessed June 10, 2018. http://plato.stanford.edu/archives/fall201/ entries/recognition/.

Jayawickrama, J. 2018. *Humanitarian Aid System is a Continuation of the Colonial Project.* Accessed September 7, 2018. https://www.aljazeera. com/indepth/opinion/humanitarian-aid-system-continuation-colonial-project-180224092528042.html.

Jeffreys, S. 2016. *Grand Hotel Abyss.* London New York: Verso.

Jennings, B. 2015. "Relational Liberty Revisited: Membership, Solidarity and a Public Health Ethics of Place." *Public Health Ethics* 8(1):7–17.

Jennings, B., and A. Dawson. 2015. "Solidarity in the Moral Imagination of Bioethics." *Hastings Center Report* 45(5):31–38.

Johnston, J. 2008. "Intellectual Property and Biomedicine." In *From Birth to Death and Bench to Clinic*: The Hastings Center Bioethics Briefing Book for Journalists, Policymakers, and Campaigns, edited by M. Crowley, 93-96. Garrison, NY: The Hastings Center.

Kamm, F. 2004. "The New Problem of Distance in Morality." In *The Ethics of Assistance*, edited by D. K. Chatterjee, 59-74. Cambridge: Cambridge University Press.

Kidd, C. 2004. "Hybridity: The Invention of Globalisation." *London Review of Books* 26(17):14–15 (14).

King, L. S. 1982. *Medical Thinking.* Princeton: Princeton University Press.

Kleinman, A. 1999. "Moral Experience and Ethical Reflection: Can Ethnography Reconcile Them? A Quandary for 'The New Bioethics'" *Daedalus* 128(4):69–97.

Kleinman, A. 2006. "Ethics and Experience: An Anthropological Approach to Health Equity." In *Public Health, Ethics, and Equity,* edited by S. Anand, F. Peter and A. Sen, 269–282. Oxford: Oxford University Press.

Kon, A. A. 2009. "The Role of Empirical Research in Bioethics." *American Journal of Bioethics* 9(6–7):59–65.

## References 189

Lackner, C., and B. Milanovic. 2013. *Global Income Distribution: From the Fall of the Berlin Wall to the Great Recession.* Accessed June 6, 2018. https://doi.org/10.1596/1813-9450-6719.

Laitinen, A., and H. Ikäheimo. 2011. *Recognition and Social Ontology.* Leiden: K. Brill NV.

Lanchester, J. 2018. "After the Fall." *London Review of Books* 5 July:3–8.

Leder, D. (ed.). 1992. *The Body in Medical Thought and Practice.* Dordrecht: Kluwer Academic Publishers.

Lehman, B. 2003. *The Pharmaceutical Industry and the Patent System.* Accessed September 27, 2018. https://users.wfu.edu/mcfallta/DIR0/pharma_patents.pdf.

Lévinas E. 1991. *Zwischen uns [Between us].* München: Karl Hanser Verlag.

Liese, B. H., N. Houghton, and L. Teplitskaya. 2014. "Development Assistance for Neglected Tropical Diseases: Progress Since 2009." *International Health* 6:162–171.

Liese, B., M. Rosenberg, and A. Schratz. 2010. "Programmes, Partnerships, and Governance for Elimination and Control of Neglected Tropical Diseases." *Lancet* 375:67–76.

Liese, B., and L. Schubert. 2009. "Official Development Assistance for Health –How Neglected are Neglected Tropical Diseases? An Analysis of Health Financing." *International Health* 1:141–47.

Luchetti, M. 2014. "Global Health and the 10/60 Gap" *British Journal of Medical Practitioners* 7(4):a731.

Lurie, P., and S. Wolfe. 1997. "Unethical Trials of Interventions to Reduce Perinatal Transmission of the Human Immunodeficiency Virus in Developing Countries." *New England Journal of Medicine* 337:853-856.

Luzzatto, L., et al. 2015. "Rare Diseases and Effective Treatment: are we Delivering?" *The Lancet* 385 (Feb. 28):750–751.

Luzzatto, L., et al. 2018. "Outrageous Prices of Orphan Drugs: A Call for Collaboration." *The Lancet.* http.//dx.doi.org/10.1016/S0140-6736(18) 1069-9.

# References

Mackey, T. K., B. A. Ling, R. Cuomo, R. Hafen, K. C. Brower, and D. E. Lee. 2014. "Emerging and Reemerging Neglected Tropical Diseases: a Review of Key Characteristics, Risk Factors, and the Policy and Innovation Environment." *Clinical Microbiology Reviews* 27(4):949–979.

Macklin, R. 2004. *Double Standards in Medical Research in Developing Countries.* Cambridge: Cambridge University Press.

Mamdani, M. 2018. "The African University." *London Review of Books* 40(14):29–32.

Marmot, M. 2018. "Just Societies, Health Equity, and Dignified Lives: the PAHO Equity Commission. *The Lancet*, September 24. http://dx.doi.org/10.1016/S0140-6736(18)32349-3.

Marshall, P. A. 1992. "Anthropology and Bioethics." *Medical Anthropology Quarterly New Series* 6(1):49–73.

Mascalzoni, D., A. Paradiso, and M. Hansson. 2014. "Rare Disease Research: Breaking the Privacy Barrier." *Applied Translational Genomics.* Accessed November 25, 2018. doi: [10.1016/j.atg.2014.04.003].

McKeown, T. 1979. *The Role of Medicine.* Oxford: Basil Blackwell.

Mercurio, B. C. 2006. "TRIPs-Plus Provisions in Ftas: Recent Trends." In *Regional Trade Agreements and the WTO Legal System*, edited by L. Bartels and F. Ortino, 215–237. Oxford: Oxford University Press. Available at SSRN: https://ssrn.com/abstract=947767.

Metha, P., and P. J. Hotez. 2016. "NTD and NCD Co-morbidities: The Example of Dengue Fever." *PLOS Neglected Tropical Diseases* August 25, 2016. Accessed September 5, 2018. doi: 10.1371/journal.pntd.0004619.

Metz, T. 2018. "How to Deal with Neglected Tropical Diseases in the Light of an African Ethic." *Developing World Bioethics* 18:233–240.

Miller, D. 1999. *Principles of Social Justice.* Cambridge, London: Harvard University Press.

Miller, D. 2004. "National Responsibility and International Justice." In *The Ethics of Assistance*, edited by D. K. Chatterjee, 123–143. Cambridge: Cambridge University Press.

## References 191

Mirowski, P., and R. Van Horn. 2005. "The Contract Research Organization and the Commercialization of Scientific Research." *Social Studies of Science* 35(4):503–548.

Molyneux, D. H., L. Savioli, and D. Engels. 2017. "Neglected Tropical Diseases: Progress towards Addressing the Chronic Pandemic." *The Lancet* 389:312–325.

Moon, S., J. Bermudez, and E. t'Hoen. 2012. "Innovation and Access to Medicines for Neglected Populations: Could a Treaty Address a Broken Pharmaceutical R&D System?" *PLoS Medicine* 9(5):1–5.

Morel, C., et al. 2007. "The Road to Recovery." *Nature* 449(13):180–182.

Moyn, S. 2018. *Not Enough. Human Rights in an Unequal World.* Cambridge: The Belknap Press.

Moynihan, R., E. Doran, and D. Henry. 2008. "Disease mongering is now part of the Global Health Debate." *PloS Medicine* 5(5): 684-686 [e106].

Muller, J. H. 1994. "Anthropology, Bioethics, and Medicine: A Provocative Trilogy." *Medical Anthropology Quarterly* 8(4):448–467.

Nutbeam, D. 2000. "Health Literacy as a Public Health Goal: a Challenge for Contemporary Health Education and Communication Strategies into the 21$^{st}$ Century." *Health Promotion International* 15(3):259–267.

Nussbaum, M. 1999. *Sex and Social Justice.* Oxford: Oxford University Press.

Nussbaum M. 2011. *Creating Capabilities.* Cambridge: The Belknap Press.

O'Connell, D. 2007. "Neglected Diseases." *Nature* 449(13):157.

O'Connell, P. 2011. "The Death of Socio-economic Rights." *The Modern Law Review* 74(4):532–554.

O'Neill, O. 2002. *A Question of Trust.* Cambridge: Cambridge University Press.

Ooms, G., and R. Hammonds. 2008. "Correcting Globalisation in Health: Transnational Entitlements versus the Ethical Imperative of Reducing Aid-dependency." *Public Health Ethics* 1(2):154–170.

Palazzo, G., F. Krings, and U. Hoffrage. 2013. "Ethical Blindness." *Journal of Business Ethics* 109(3):323–338.

## References

Petersen, A., and D. Lupton. 2000. *The New Public Health*. London: SAGE Publications.

Petryna, A. 2007. "Clinical Trials Offshored: On Private Sector Science and Public Health." *BioSocieties* 2:21–40.

Ploumen, L., and E. Schippers. 2017. "Better Life Through Medicine – Let's Leave No One Behind. *The Lancet* 389(10067):339–341.

Pogge, T. 2008. "Access to Medicines." *Public Health Ethics* 1(2):73–82.

Pogge, T. 2009. "The Health Impact Fund and Its Justification by Appeal to Human Rights." *Journal of Social Philosophy* 49(2):542–569.

Porter, B. 2015. "*Background Paper for a Presentation to the Continuing Committee of Officials on Human Rights.*" Accessed September 30, 2018. http://www.socialrights.ca/documents/publications/Porter%20 Progressive%20Implementation.pdf.

Potter, V. R. 1971. *BIOETHICS Bridge to the Future*. Englewood Cliffs: Prentice-Hall.

Ramsay, S. 2001. "No Closure in Sight for the 10/90 Health-research Gap." *The Lancet* 358 (October 20):1348.

Reich, W. T. 1995. "The World 'Bioethics': The Struggle Over its Earliest Meanings." *Kennedy Institute of Ethics Journal* 5(1):19–34.

Reid-Henry, S. 2013. "Review Essay: On the Politics of our Humanitarian Present." *Environment and Planning D: Society and Space* 31:753–760.

Ridley, B., H. G. Grabowski, and J. L. Moe. 2006. "Developing Drugs for Developing Countries." *Health Affairs* 25(2):313–324.

Roos, R. A. C. 2010. "Huntington's Disease: Clinical Review." *Orphanet Journal of Rare Diseases*. Accessed May 10, 2018. https://doi.org/ 10.1186/1750-1172-5-40.

Sachs, J. D. 2012. "From Millennium Development Goals to Sustainable Development Goals." *The Lancet*. Accessed August 29, 2018. doi: https://doi.org/10.1016/S0140-6736(12)60685-0.

Sass, H-M. 2007. "Fritz Jahr's 1927 Concept of Bioethics." *Kennedy Institute of Ethics Journal* 17(4):279–295.

Sastya, S., V. Karunakaran, N. Muwel, C. Chandrakanta, and N. Jamra. 2018. "Neglected Parasitic Infections (NPIs) of Tropical Countries:

# References 193

Current Status and Control Strategies." *Journal of Entomology and Zoology Studies* 6(4):265–270.

Savulescu, J. 2006. "Conscientious Objection in Medicine." *British Medical Journal*. doi: 10.1136/bmj.332.7536.294.

Schuck, M. J. 1991. *That They Be One*. Washington D.C.: Georgetown University Press.

Selgelid, M. J. 2008. "A Full-Pull Program for the Provision of Pharmaceuticals: Practical Issues." *Public Health Ethics* 1(2):134–145.

Shue, H. 2004. "Thickening Convergence: Human Rights and Cultural Diversity." In *The Ethics of Assistance*, edited by D. K. Chatterjee, 217-241. Cambridge: Cambridge University Press.

Sen, A. 1995. *Inequality Reexamined*. Cambridge: Harvard University Press.

Singer, P. 1972. "Famine, Affluence, and Morality." *Philosophy and Public Affairs* 1(3):229–243.

Singer, P. 1972. "Famine, Affluence, and Morality." *Philosophy and Public Affairs* 1(3):229–243.

Singer, P. 2004. "Outsiders: Our Obligations to Those Beyond Our Borders." In *The Ethics of Assistance*, edited by D. K. Chatterjee DK, 11-32. Cambridge: Cambridge University Press.

Singer, P. 2015. "Life-saving Drugs for All." *Project Syndicate*, May 12.

Singer, P. A. 2007. "A Tough Transition." *Nature* 449(13):160–163. Accessed June 9, 2018. https://www.project-syndicate.org/commentary /drugs-investment-developing-countries-by-peter-singer-2015-05.

Sontag, S. 2003. *Regarding the Pain of Others*. New York: Picador.

Stafford, M., C. von Wagner, S. Perman, J. Taylor, D. Kuh, and J. Sherringham. 2018. "Social Connectedness and Engagement in Preventive Health Services: An Analysis of Data from a Prospective Cohort Study." *Lancet Public Health*. doi: http://dx.doi.org/10.1016/ S2468-2667(18)30141-5.

Taylor, C. 1995. *Philosophical Arguments*. Cambridge London: Harvard University Press.

ten Have, H. 2015. "Bioethics Needs Bayonets." In *Global Ethics: What For?* edited by G. Solinis, 147-150. Paris: UNESCO.

Theobald, S., et al. 2018. "*Implementation Research: New Imperatives and Opportunities in Global Health.*" doi.org/10.1016/S0140-6736(18) 32205-0.

Toulmin, S. 1997. "How Medicine Saved the Life of Ethics." In *Bioethics: An Introduction to the History, Methods, and Practice*, edited by N. S. Jecker, A. R. Jonsen, and R. A. Pearlman, 26–34. London: Jones and Bartlett Publishers, Inc.

Turner, L. 2007. "Global Health Inequalities and Bioethics." In *The Ethics of Bioethics*, edited by L. A. Eckenwiller, and F. G. Cohn, 229-240. Baltimore: The Johns Hopkins University Press.

Turner, L. 2009. "Anthropological and Sociological Critiques of Bioethics." *Bioethical Inquiry* 6:83–98.

Vetter, M. 2008. "Natality and Biopolitics in Hannah Arendt." *Revista de Ciencia Política* 28(2):137–159.

Wenner, D. M. 2017. "The Social Value of Knowledge and Responsiveness." *Bioethics* 31(2):97–104.

Wieland, W. 1975. *Diagnose. Überlegungen zur Medizintheorie [Diagnosis. Reflections on Medical Theory]*. Berlin: Walter de Gruyter.

White, S. 2015. "*Social Minimum.*" Stanford Encyclopedia of Philosophy. Accessed August 31, 2018. http://plato.stanford.edu/archives/win2015/entries/social-minimum/.

WHO. 1986. "*Ottawa Charter for Health Promotion.*" Accessed May 28, 2018. www.euro.who.int/__data/assets/pdf_file/.../Ottawa_Charter.pdf.

WHO. 2009. Accessed August 18, 2018. http://www.who.int/neglected_diseases/Human_rights_approach_to_NTD_Eng_ok.pdf.

Young, R., T. Bekele, A. Gunn, et al. 2018. "Developing New Health Technologies for Neglected Diseases: A Pipeline Portfolio Review and Cost Model [version 2; referees: 2 approved, 1 approved with reservations]. *Gates Open Res.* Accessed September 7, 2018. doi: 10.12688/gatesopenres.12817.2.

Yuthavong, Y. 2015. "Future Trends in Bioscience and Biotechnology and their Ethical Consideration." In *Global Ethics: What for?* edited by G. Solinis, 121-124. Paris: UNESCO 2015.

## References

Zwart, H., L. Landeweerd, and A. van Rooij. 2014. "Adapt or Perish: Assessing the Recent Shift in the European Research Funding Arena from 'ELSA' to 'RRI'." *Life Sciences, Society and Policy* 24:11–30.

# ABOUT THE AUTHOR

## Miguel Kottow, MD
Full Professor
Faculty of Medicine, Universidad de Chile, Santiago, Chile
Email: mkottow@gmail.com

Miguel Kottow, born in Israel (1939) and raised in Chile, where he studied medicine at the Universidad Chile. Specialized in ophthalmology, he has practiced in public healthcare institutions and private practice. Since his graduation, he has been on the faculty staff of the Faculty of Medicine, Universidad de Chile where he became Full Professor (1993). Doctor of Medicine (Bonn, Germany) and Master's degree in Sociology (Hagen, Germany). Actively engaged in bioethics, and focusing on public health bioethics, Kottow has taught in medical schools at graduate and post-graduate level in Chile and other Latin American countries. Numerous publications of articles, books and encyclopedia contributions, as well as single authored books on ophthalmology, bioethics, medicine and philosophy, including "From Justice to Protection" (Springer 2012), "Towards a Medical Anthropology of Ageing" (CSP, 2017), "Desde la Bioética: comienzo y final del cuerpo humano" (Ed. Universitaria, 2016). He lives in Santiago, Chile.

# INDEX

## #

10/90 gap, 60, 65, 66

## A

absolute poverty, xiii, 9, 10, 77, 110, 125
activism, 27, 161, 178
acute infection, 87
Africa, 14, 31, 66, 75, 88
AIDS, 14, 81, 153
amyotrophic lateral sclerosis, 90
anthrax, 82, 83
anthropological features, 97, 103, 105, 109, 110, 164
anthropology, vii, 97, 98, 99, 102, 110, 111, 132, 161, 190, 191, 197
antibiotic, 121
antivenom, 83
antiviral agents, 35
aspirational ethics, 68, 69
atrocities, 1, 100, 175
authoritarianism, 159

## B

basic needs, xiii, 17, 18, 22, 23, 38, 125, 127, 175
benefits, xi, 8, 15, 23, 24, 49, 51, 52, 53, 56, 60, 65, 69, 80, 122, 126, 150, 151, 152, 165, 168
biobanks, 56, 57
biodiversity, 112, 113, 116, 182
bioethics, xi, xii, 7, 8, 51, 58, 97, 98, 102, 103, 113, 119, 130, 133, 139, 143, 144, 145, 146, 147, 148, 149, 150, 151, 152, 153, 154, 155, 156, 157, 158, 159, 160, 161, 162, 163, 164, 166, 167, 168, 169, 171, 177, 178, 187, 197
biological processes, 35
biomedical innovations, 148
biomedical knowledge, 42
biomedicalization, 42, 183
biomedicine, 41, 42, 48, 50, 143, 148, 155, 161, 183, 188
biopolitics, 17, 194
biopower, 17, 141
biotechnology, 48, 143, 147, 151
black market, 33

## 200    Index

blue marble, 83, 84, 88, 89, 125, 132, 169, 187
Bolivia, 69
Brazil, 31, 41, 62, 88, 90, 184
Britain, 41, 49, 84

## C

capability, 23, 29, 30, 32, 39
capacity building, 85
capitalism, ix, 19, 26, 34, 100, 107, 141, 153, 171
Chagas disease, 83, 87, 89
Chile, 197
China, 10, 66, 90, 141
Christianity, 185
clinical encounter, 39, 40, 42
clinical trials, 50, 52, 53, 58, 60, 67, 69, 93, 167
common morality, 145, 159, 185
Contract Research Organizations (CROs), 53, 56, 58, 59, 60, 67, 68, 126, 156
control group, 52, 68, 69, 157
cost, 17, 43, 44, 49, 57, 58, 59, 60, 61, 65, 74, 75, 83, 93, 94, 112, 122, 127, 130, 136, 137, 169
cost saving, 59
cultural values, 97, 154
culture, 7, 9, 26, 40, 49, 73, 84, 97, 98, 99, 101, 103, 105, 107, 109, 151

## D

developed countries, 49, 67, 74, 91, 121
developed nations, 69
developing countries, 64, 75, 133, 135, 136, 137, 167
developing world, 69, 101, 182, 184, 190
development assistance, xii, 10, 173
developmental process, 104
diabetes, 87

dignity, xii, 1, 2, 7, 8, 19, 25, 33, 76, 99, 102, 104, 119, 145
disability, 9, 36, 37, 81, 83
disaster, 146
discomfort, 125, 153
discourse ethics, 116
discrimination, 22, 24, 27, 28, 29, 30, 47, 75, 84, 130, 131, 144, 152, 160, 161
disease, vii, xiii, 4, 8, 9, 10, 14, 31, 35, 36, 37, 38, 39, 40, 42, 43, 44, 45, 49, 54, 56, 57, 58, 59, 65, 66, 75, 79, 80, 81, 82, 83, 86, 87, 89, 91, 93, 94, 98, 123, 124, 126, 134, 145, 147, 150, 163, 173, 178, 187, 190, 191, 192
disease mongering, 36, 42, 43, 44, 45, 66, 126, 191
diseases, x, xi, xiii, 8, 13, 14, 35, 36, 38, 39, 41, 42, 43, 45, 49, 50, 53, 55, 56, 57, 59, 60, 66, 73, 74, 75, 76, 77, 81, 82, 83, 84, 85, 86, 87, 89, 90, 91, 92, 93, 94, 106, 119, 120, 121, 122, 123, 124, 125, 126, 127, 128, 129, 130, 131, 132, 133, 135, 137, 139, 147, 150, 151, 153, 157, 158, 160, 166, 169, 171, 172, 173, 175, 194
distributive justice, 19, 24, 25, 152
diversity, xi, 22, 98, 120, 140, 178
DOHA, 61, 62, 65, 126, 176, 184
drug companies, 16, 54, 67, 73, 94, 153, 181
drugs, 8, 16, 41, 43, 49, 50, 54, 55, 56, 57, 59, 60, 61, 62, 64, 65, 66, 67, 68, 72, 75, 80, 82, 84, 87, 88, 89, 90, 91, 92, 93, 94, 121, 133, 137, 166, 193
Drugs for Neglected Diseases Initiative (DNDI), 84, 137

## E

economic assistance, xii
economic development, 10, 61, 130, 131
economic growth, 130
economic incentives, 94

## Index

economic independence, 61
economic power, 21, 176
economic values, 24
economics, 4, 9, 17, 57, 58, 158, 163, 172
education, 9, 13, 74, 77, 79, 90, 120, 130
educational attainment, 89
educational opportunities, 17
egalitarianism, 20
elderly population, 25
embryonic stem cells, 60
emerging infectious diseases, 76
employment, 9, 27, 126, 157
empowerment, 11, 13, 20, 23, 30, 32, 33,
    37, 77, 79, 85, 110, 126, 140, 141, 159,
    161, 165
energy, 11, 18, 77, 100, 138
environmental change, 178
environmental degradation, 10, 15
environmental factors, 36
environmental sustainability, 10
epidemic, xii, 14, 55, 63, 121, 124, 150, 173
epidemiology, 38
epidermolysis bullosa, 54
ethical issues, 119, 146, 154
ethical standards, 51, 67, 69
ethics, x, xi, xii, 4, 7, 16, 21, 26, 29, 30, 33,
    35, 41, 45, 47, 48, 51, 52, 54, 60, 66, 68,
    69, 71, 72, 97, 100, 105, 106, 111, 112,
    115, 116, 122, 128, 129, 139, 143, 144,
    145, 146, 148, 149, 150, 151, 152, 154,
    155, 156, 157, 158, 159, 163, 164, 167,
    171, 174, 175, 176, 177
ethics committees, 51, 68
ethics of recognition, 26, 29, 30, 33
ethnic culture, 109
ethnographers, 162
eugenics, 144, 154
Europe, 66, 88, 94
European Community, 93
European Union, 11, 91
euthanasia, 144, 161
everyday life, 37, 160, 165

exclusion, 14, 16, 30, 65, 95, 100, 141, 165
expenditures, 55, 65, 90
exploitation, 14, 34, 51, 73, 100, 136, 140,
    144, 152
extreme poverty, 9, 10, 77, 138

## F

fairness, xi, 21, 25, 63, 78, 79, 127, 145,
    154, 165, 166
famine, 6, 132, 138, 139
fanaticism, 100
food, 9, 11, 16, 23, 82, 89, 105, 126, 149,
    152
Food and Drug Administration (FDA), 44,
    68, 69, 92, 94, 134
food production, 16, 149
food security, 9
force, ix, 27, 78, 100, 107, 118, 127
Free Trade Agreements (FTAs), 62, 63,
    126, 176
future generations, 18, 147, 154

## G

gender inequality, 10, 26
gene therapy, 54
genes, 38, 48
genetic alteration, 38
genetic defect, 56
genetic disease, 93
genetic engineering, 149
genetics, 9, 38, 102, 128, 144, 149, 155,
    156, 157
genome, 38
genomics, 149, 151
Germany, 15, 197
global health, 14, 56, 66, 83, 86, 127, 129,
    136, 154, 182, 186, 187, 189, 191, 194
global inequality, 10

## 202 *Index*

globalization, xi, 3, 9, 15, 16, 17, 19, 20, 27, 86, 88, 124, 125, 130, 131, 132, 133, 141, 147, 151, 152, 153, 171, 172, 173

God, 19, 99, 100, 178

goods and services, 15, 18, 20, 25, 88, 116

governments, 16, 37, 49, 57, 88, 134, 135, 136, 157

Gulf Coast, 89, 187

### H

H1N1 flu, 153

health, vii, xi, xii, 3, 6, 7, 9, 13, 14, 16, 21, 22, 23, 25, 35, 36, 37, 38, 39, 40, 41, 42, 43, 44, 53, 54, 55, 57, 58, 59, 62, 65, 66, 68, 72, 73, 74, 75, 77, 78, 79, 80, 82, 83, 84, 85, 86, 87, 88, 89, 90, 93, 101, 117, 121, 122, 123, 124, 125, 126, 127, 129, 130, 131, 134, 135, 136, 137, 145, 146, 147, 150, 151, 153, 154, 155, 158, 159, 161, 163, 165, 167, 169, 172, 173, 175, 177, 178, 181, 182, 183, 184, 185, 186, 187, 188, 189, 190, 191, 192, 193, 194, 197

health care, 88, 129, 130, 131, 151, 163

health condition, 83, 89, 167

health education, 42

health problems, 14, 86, 150, 161

health promotion, 37, 42

health services, 41, 74, 117, 131

healthcare, x, xi, xii, xiii, 3, 6, 9, 10, 14, 15, 23, 25, 26, 33, 35, 36, 38, 39, 40, 41, 42, 49, 55, 57, 59, 62, 66, 67, 69, 72, 73, 78, 79, 80, 83, 84, 87, 88, 89, 90, 91, 93, 94, 118, 120, 121, 122, 124, 125, 126, 127, 129, 131, 135, 136, 138, 144, 145, 148, 150, 151, 153, 155, 159, 161, 164, 165, 166, 168, 169, 171, 172, 173, 174, 175, 177, 178

healthism, 38, 40

HIV

HIV/AIDS, xii, 14, 55, 69, 81, 83, 86, 87, 125, 153, 154

human dignity, 31, 33, 118

human nature, 98, 102, 111, 115, 116, 144

human right(s), xii, 1, 2, 4, 5, 6, 7, 16, 20, 25, 45, 73, 78, 79, 102, 128, 129, 130, 131, 133, 136, 151, 162, 177, 181, 185, 186, 187, 191, 192, 193

human subjects, 51, 167

human values, 51, 143

humanitarian aid, ix, 12, 85

humanitarian intervention, 132

humanitarianism, 133, 175

### I

identity, 5, 27, 28, 29, 30, 31, 32, 40, 79, 103, 105, 106, 108, 109, 117, 164, 165, 174, 182

illness, 9, 39, 40, 41, 43, 97, 183

immunization, 12, 122

income, ix, 9, 10, 11, 18, 23, 33, 36, 49, 50, 61, 62, 66, 67, 68, 73, 75, 77, 78, 79, 82, 85, 88, 91, 120, 130, 132, 134, 135, 138, 139, 141, 150, 161, 167, 168, 173

income inequality, 141

India, 10, 12, 31, 62, 66, 90

individual rights, 16, 68

individualism, 102, 118, 119

individuality, 5, 32, 79, 108, 109, 117

individuals, 13, 23, 27, 28, 29, 30, 42, 52, 79, 104, 118, 127, 134, 137, 150, 154, 162, 164, 165, 168, 172, 177

indoctrination, 103

industries, 126, 156, 157, 168, 169

industry, 8, 42, 43, 44, 50, 53, 54, 55, 56, 57, 58, 59, 61, 63, 64, 65, 67, 69, 75, 84, 94, 120, 134, 136, 137, 146, 147, 148, 151, 155, 156, 167, 169, 176, 177

inequality, xii, 10, 16, 17, 20, 21, 24, 47, 80, 124, 125, 127, 130, 150, 152, 153, 178

## Index

inequity, x, xiii, 7, 9, 16, 66, 78, 80, 88, 109, 140, 152, 153, 175, 176, 177
infection, 14, 87, 124, 153
infectious agents, 14
infectious diseases, 35, 36, 74, 77, 82, 86, 121, 123, 132, 153, 171, 173
informed consent, 51, 52, 53, 68, 148, 167, 168
infrastructure, 61, 67, 88
insecurity, 77, 89, 125, 138
Institutional Review Boards, 58, 185
institutions, 11, 15, 22, 28, 41, 49, 50, 106, 131, 155, 167, 197
International Covenant on Civil and Political Rights, 78
International Covenant on Economic, Social and Cultural Rights, 3, 8
International Monetary Fund, 15, 41
investment, 73, 81, 85, 94, 133, 135, 168, 193
Israel, 174, 177, 197

### L

Latin America, 66, 67, 68, 186, 197
LDCs, 61, 62
Least Developed Countries (LDCs), 61, 62
leprosy, 84
liberty, 2, 32, 107, 115
life expectancy, 79, 121, 154
life sciences, 128, 144, 157, 159
lifestyle changes, 15
living conditions, 80, 125
low-income poverty, 77

### M

malaria, 81, 86, 90, 154
malnutrition, 6, 16, 154
maltreatment, 25
man-made disasters, 115

marginalization, 24, 28, 100, 106, 152, 165
market economy, x, 26, 153, 155, 179
marketing, 15, 41, 44, 56, 59, 65, 93, 94, 145, 156
Médecins Sans Frontières, 84, 127, 132
medical care, 13, 39, 42, 44, 53, 79, 85, 90, 91, 97, 145, 159, 161
medicalization, x, 36, 38, 39, 40, 41, 42, 43, 44, 45, 66, 80, 121, 125, 175, 184
medication, 9, 18, 44, 64, 67, 74, 80, 84, 87, 121, 137, 153
medicine, xi, 14, 35, 36, 38, 41, 42, 43, 48, 49, 54, 56, 59, 66, 84, 100, 102, 121, 126, 143, 145, 150, 154, 159, 169, 175, 176, 177, 197
Medicine Patent Pool (MPP), 137
me-too drugs, 66
Mexico, 127
microorganisms, 13, 35, 173
migrants, 5, 26, 29, 141, 162
migration, 79
military, ix, 14, 131
minorities, 24, 26, 27, 39, 66, 160
misdistribution, 24
mission, 84, 158
morality, 20, 28, 29, 72, 115, 116, 144, 145, 159, 164, 174
mundane transcendence, 105, 107, 110

### N

neglect, x, 16, 25, 30, 33, 36, 71, 72, 73, 75, 76, 77, 79, 80, 82, 88, 89, 91, 93, 100, 116, 119, 120, 122, 125, 131, 133, 134, 135, 140, 141, 145, 151, 153, 155, 164, 166, 168, 169, 171, 175, 177, 179, 184
neglected populations, vii, xi, 5, 23, 37, 40, 41, 66, 76, 117, 125, 130, 131, 139, 162, 165, 168, 169, 191
neoliberal globalization, 9, 17, 19, 130, 152, 153

# 204 *Index*

non-communicable diseases, 36
non-profitable drugs, 92

## O

off-shoring, 167
Organization for Economic Co-operation
and Development (OECD), 11, 56
orphan drugs, 8, 55, 57, 60, 64, 65, 92, 93,
181, 187, 189
outsourcing, 59, 60, 67, 69

## P

participative parity, 26, 27
patents, 49, 50, 54, 55, 59, 60, 61, 62, 63,
64, 66, 67, 134, 153, 168, 189
personal identity, 28, 29, 30, 105, 164
pharma industry, 54, 55, 56, 61, 63, 65, 67,
137, 176
pharmaceutical, 8, 42, 43, 49, 50, 53, 55, 56,
58, 59, 60, 61, 64, 67, 69, 74, 75, 84, 92,
93, 94, 120, 121, 123, 126, 135, 136,
137, 151, 155, 156, 157, 168, 169, 177,
178
phocomelia, 92
placebos, 52, 53, 54, 68, 69, 157
poverty, xiii, 8, 9, 10, 11, 13, 14, 19, 20, 22,
25, 33, 43, 73, 74, 75, 77, 79, 81, 83, 86,
88, 89, 90, 110, 119, 121, 122, 123, 124,
125, 140, 141, 151, 169, 171
poverty line, 11, 33, 89
public health, xi, 8, 13, 14, 35, 38, 41, 42,
43, 44, 62, 65, 72, 74, 75, 80, 82, 84, 85,
86, 87, 90, 121, 123, 124, 126, 127, 129,
133, 145, 146, 147, 149, 150, 153, 154,
155, 158, 159, 161, 165, 169, 175, 177,
178, 181, 182, 184, 186, 188, 191, 192,
193, 197
public health ethics, 154, 186, 188, 191,
192, 193

## Q

qualitative research, 51
quality of life, 102, 112, 130
quality standards, 59

## R

race, 24, 27, 65
racism, 160
randomized clinical trial, 68
rare diseases, vii, x, xi, 49, 53, 55, 56, 57,
59, 60, 66, 71, 75, 82, 90, 91, 92, 93, 94,
121, 122, 128, 160, 166, 169, 181, 182,
183, 185, 186, 187, 188, 189, 192
rationing, 65, 159
recognition, 2, 9, 13, 25, 26, 27, 28, 29, 30,
31, 32, 33, 80, 84, 105, 106, 127, 147,
164, 165, 171, 183, 185, 188, 189
redistribution, 23, 24, 25, 26, 29, 30, 127,
relationality, 31, 105, 106, 107, 110
relative poverty, xiii, 10, 22, 43, 77, 125
research and development, 55, 56, 82, 84,
120
resources, x, xi, xii, 3, 17, 18, 22, 25, 27, 37,
44, 57, 63, 65, 66, 69, 73, 78, 82, 123,
124, 125, 126, 131, 152, 159, 163, 173
right to health, 6, 7, 38, 39, 78, 130, 131,
139
rights, 1, 2, 3, 4, 5, 6, 7, 25, 26, 28, 29, 31,
32, 55, 60, 76, 78, 79, 99, 104, 129, 130,
131, 134, 136, 140, 164, 167, 171, 183,
194
risk epidemiology, 38

## S

Site Management Organizations (SMOs), 58
social empowerment, 33, 110
social environment, 23, 42, 150

## Index

social inequalities, 13
social institutions, 47, 117
social integration, 17, 22, 24, 29, 105
social justice, 19, 20, 26, 28, 30
social market economy, 19
social minimum, 12, 20, 22, 23, 194
social movements, 26, 160
social order, 66, 106, 139
social organization, 106
social participation, 30
social problems, 145, 147
social relations, 108, 145
social responsibility, 8, 60, 167, 169
social structure, 28, 163
social welfare, 16, 126
society, ix, 4, 21, 22, 24, 26, 28, 32, 47, 48, 49, 103, 105, 116, 127, 128, 139, 147, 148, 158
solidarity, xii, 12, 16, 28, 29, 76, 107, 117, 118, 119, 129, 139, 153, 154, 186, 188
South Africa, 49, 137
sustainability, 10, 12, 17, 18, 113, 147
sustainable development, 10, 11. 17, 86, 137, 192
sustainable growth, 24, 111, 151, 154

### T

technoscience, 47, 48, 99, 147
thalidomide, 92
The World Trade Organization (WTO), 61, 190
therapeutic agents, x, 56, 67, 82, 90, 93, 176

therapeutic approaches, 56
therapeutics, 126
Trade-related Aspects of Intellectual Property Rights (TRIPs), 61, 62, 63, 126, 176, 190
transcendence of the self, 105, 109
tuberculosis, 8, 13, 80, 81, 86, 154
typhus, 82, 89

### U

UNESCO, 7, 8, 157, 162, 177, 178, 181, 194, 195
Universal Declaration of Human Rights, 1, 2

### V

vaccines, 8, 49, 50, 55, 64, 75, 82, 84, 85, 87, 88, 89, 121, 134, 135, 137, 153, 165
vested interests, 40, 53, 149, 161, 166
voluntary organizations, 37

### W

World Health Organization (WHO), xi, 9, 12, 14, 36, 37, 42, 43, 73, 74, 75, 78, 83, 87, 122, 127, 129, 130, 131, 153, 184, 187, 194
World Trade Organization (WTO), 61, 190

# Related Nova Publications

## BIOETHICS: ISSUES AND DILEMMAS

**EDITOR:** Tyler N. Pace

**SERIES:** Ethical Issues in the 21st Century

**BOOK DESCRIPTION:** This new book presents research in the expansive field of bioethics including biomedical ethics in obstetrics, ethical decision making in the health care system, the feasibility of using human oocytes for stem cell research, as well as mandatory circumcision in Sub-Saharan Africa to prevent HIV and AIDS and environmental ethics to preserve the world for future generations.

**HARDCOVER ISBN:** 978-1-61728-290-4
**RETAIL PRICE:** $130

## DISEASES, DRUGS AND QUALITY OF LIFE

**AUTHOR:** Marwan S.M. Al-Nimer

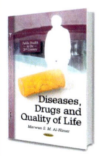

**SERIES:** Public Health in the 21st Century

**BOOK DESCRIPTION:** This book presents current research in health-related quality of life, with a particular focus on disease and drugs.

**HARDCOVER ISBN:** 978-1-62100-130-0
**RETAIL PRICE:** $87

To see complete list of Nova publications, please visit our website at www.novapublishers.com

# Related Nova Publications

## HUMAN DIGNITY AND BIOETHICS

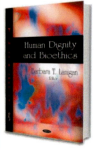

EDITOR: Barbara T. Lanigan

BOOK DESCRIPTION: The book will explore some of the complex roots of the modern notion of human dignity, in order to shed light on why its application to bioethics is so problematic. Finally, it will suggest, tentatively, that a certain conception of human dignity—dignity understood as humanity— has an important role to play in bioethics, both now and especially in the future.

HARDCOVER ISBN: 978-1-60692-470-9
RETAIL PRICE: $215

## BIOETHICS: SELECT LAWS AND ISSUES FROM AROUND THE WORLD

EDITORS: Marshall Breslau and Paige Feldman

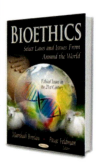

SERIES: Ethical Issues in the 21st Century

BOOK DESCRIPTION: This book examines the field of bioethics from an international and regional legal perspective. It focuses on major international law documents such as the United Nations Universal Declaration on Bioethics and Human Rights and UNESCO declarations on human cloning and the human genome.

SOFTCOVER ISBN: 978-1-62948-280-4
RETAIL PRICE: $58

To see complete list of Nova publications, please visit our website at www.novapublishers.com